The Testosterone
Syndrome

THE TESTOSTERONE SYNDROME

The Critical Factor for Energy, Health, and Sexuality— Reversing the Male Menopause

EUGENE SHIPPEN, M.D., AND WILLIAM FRYER

❏

M. Evans and Company, Inc.
New York

M. Evans and Company, Inc.
216 East 49th Street
New York, New York 10017

Library of Congress Cataloging-in-Publication Data

Shippen, Eugene.
    The testosterone syndrome : the critical factor for energy, health, and sexuality—reversing the male menopause / Eugene Shippen and William Fryer.
        p.   cm.
    Includes index.
    ISBN 0-87131-829-6 (cloth)
    1. Tesosterone—Therapeutic use.   2. Climacteric, Male—Hormone therapy. I. Fryer, William, 1949-   . II. Title.
    RC884.S55 1998
    615'.366—dc21   97-43349

DESIGN AND TYPESETTING BY RIK LAIN SCHELL

Manufactured in the United States of America

9 8 7 6 5 4 3 2 1

Contents

Preface

If I told you that one key substance in the body is more powerful than any other health factor, is more closely linked to risk of illness if and when a deficiency occurs, is more misunderstood, more improperly used, and more tragically underused than any other, what would it be? Testosterone! I have studied it, prescribed it, and watched the responses of my patients—hundreds of them. I challenge anyone to find a more diversely positive factor in men's health. When normally abundant, it is at the core of energy, strength, stamina, and sexuality. When deficient, it is at the core of disease and early demise.

Testosterone deficiency has been an unrecognized syndrome that impacts every sinew and cell in the body. It is powerfully linked to nearly every major degenerative disease. Use of this remarkable healing hormone could reverse suffering and prevent early death. My research uncovered a mountain of medical literature that has been basically ignored supporting its benefits.

I was taught that there was no male menopause and for years accepted that as fact. A series of events in my own health and the discovery that several pioneering physicians held entirely differing points of view changed my mind and transformed my conception of age-related illness and preventive medicine. Until that point, I had seen aging as an unrelenting natural process that it was best to accept gracefully. Preventive medicine was an attempt to treat or modify specific risk factors that, like a sleeping lion, would jump up and bite you later in life.

My perspective changed dramatically. Clearly, preventive medicine would widen in scope if it turned out aging was reversible. And, to a significant extent, it is. The male menopause, a grim milestone in the middle passage of a man's life, can be rolled back.

Testosterone decline is at the core of that male menopause (and a key element in the female menopause as well). Naturally, the two sexes have a different experience of midlife menopausal change. In women, there is an explosion of in-your-face symptoms, while men's very similar symptoms sneak in the back door unexpectedly like a thief in the night. Too often, loss of energy, ambition, sexual drive, and a host of minor symptoms are written off as "burnout" or depression.

Women, meanwhile, have already learned that hormone replacement results in reversal of the physical changes of menopause. Men, confronted by an information vacuum, still need to make the same discovery.

There are, of course, scientists on both sides of the fence. Even after forty years of experience, few subjects engender more emotion and controversy than estrogen replacement for women. Yet the vast majority of studies show a risk-benefit ratio that emphatically favors the camp of hormonal replacement. The considerable literature on testosterone replacement shows a very similar balance of benefit over risk. Keep that in mind and remember that quality of life is clearly the cornerstone of all treatment decisions.

Why have the subject of male menopause and the advantages of testosterone therapy taken so long to surface? One can only speculate. Perhaps the unspeakable spectre of impotence is at the root of silence. Perhaps it simply takes time for new ideas to rise into the medical mainstream. Old dogmas and clinical habits die hard. It is well for us not to rashly assume that every new nostrum has value, but resistence in the face of overwhelming science has no excuse. To prevent the suffering of many is, for me, a powerful motivator. That is why I wrote this book.

Resistance will fade. Testosterone therapy has every prospect of becoming for men what estrogen therapy is now for millions of women. The male menopause, a real tragedy in the midlife of the average man, has had its day. I am going to put a stake through its ugly little heart. I promise.

—Eugene R. Shippen, M.D.

CHAPTER 1:

A Menopause for Men

A menopause for men? You'd better believe it. Men are in no way immune to midlife changes. They, too, suffer those transforming physical experiences that—when we see them in women—we call, with definitive finality, the *change of life*. It's the big change—the one that means you're no longer young.

Of course, we all change constantly as the years tick by. We get used to it. The alterations in our physical identity seem familiar, expected, even comfortable. But then suddenly, at some point in our lives, we are genuinely startled. Changes occur that we hadn't bargained for. Aging no longer looks benign. Pain, weariness, the fraying of desire, the dark shadow of depression—all proclaim that a toll is being taken on our bodies and our spirits. By and large, the toll gates of change are hormonal. For some, the price of entry will be very high indeed.

Surely it makes sense to ask whether we can't reverse some part of this process of aging. Would it surprise you to know we can?

Allow me to define a word, without which the rest of this book is meaningless. *Hormone.* A hormone is a chemical substance produced in one part or organ of the body that starts or runs the activity of an organ or a group of cells in another part of the body. Testosterone, estrogen, insulin, adrenalin, cortisone—these are a few of the hormones found in most people's vocabularies and at least vaguely understood. Hormones can also be converted from one hormonal substance into another out in the tissues of the body. This is a newer concept, which later in the book will prove vital, and it is referred to as intracrinology.

In the last few years, the popular anti-aging literature has given many people a familiarity with such hormones as DHEA, growth hormone, and melatonin. They are genuinely important substances, and perhaps some of you are already familiar with the idea that the levels of hormones can affect our actual (as opposed to chronological) rate of aging.

Every cell in the body is programmed by hormonal messengers. Hormones tune our systems—or untune them. We are hormonal creatures to at least as great an extent as we are oxygen-breathing creatures or blood-circulating creatures. We could not live a day or hardly even an hour without properly balanced hormonal input. Balance is the crucial word. Too much of the more important hormones would burn us out metabolically at a fantastic rate. Too little and our systems begin to slowly shut down.

Think back to when you were young. If you were like most people, you reached your physical peak in your late teens or early twenties. It was a time of rambunctious energy that resisted every effort to squander it away. Late nights, too much work and too much play, and, for many of us, far too much eating and drinking—all this produced very little in the way of untoward effects. For many twenty-year-olds, burning the candle at both ends is not a danger; it's an art form. Pushing past every reasonable limit, we recharged our cellular batteries as fast as we drained them. How were our organ systems and, indeed, every cell in our bodies able to keep up with the brutal pace? Hormones! We were in hormone heaven.

The optimal function of every cell requires optimal hormonal input—and we had it. Logically, therefore, any decline in hormonal activity from youthful norms will result in suboptimal cellular activity. Does that seem reasonable?

We know that it is. There are many reasons hormones change, including illness, stress, the autoimmune destruction of our glands, and, of course, the natural decline of aging. Any doctor who has carefully charted the hormonal changes of his patients knows that significant, long-term hormonal decline leads irresistibly toward illness, fatigue, malaise, and further aging.

And any doctor who looks for hormonal decline will find hormonal decline. Most of the major hormone systems drop significantly and steadily from year to year and decade to decade. It is one of the most important parts of the steady downward spiral into old age and debility.

Yet, incredibly, these major hormones can—so far as I know, without exception—be safely and efficiently replaced in men's and women's bodies. The result of that replacement is rapid improvement in physical function. More often than not, there is also a marked recovery in psychological attitude and mental alertness. This is a fact not widely known to laypeople and still stoutly resisted by some members of the medical profession.

The major controversy among physicians is whether gradual hormonal decline is a normal, healthy part of aging or is a pathologic, disease-like state. To me, this controversy sets up a false dichotomy. Hormonal decline is, of course, normal, but so is heart disease. They are also—and equally—disease states and will, in the end, prove fatal to any human being who allows either one to run its course unhindered.

Fortunately, the notion of hormone replacement is already well established in one corner of medical practice. I'm referring, of course, to estrogen replacement therapy for post-menopausal women. Some would suggest that this is quite different from giving testosterone to a man. Women have a menopause. Men obviously do not.

But didn't we just say that wasn't true? You're absolutely right!

Men Are Different from Women

Habitual knee-jerk reactions often go by the name of thought, and many people "think" that there is no male menopause. Why do they think this? Because an assumption is made that if a man had a menopause, it would conform to the pattern experienced by women. And, in women, menopause is anything but quiet. The cymbals clash, the hot flashes rush in, hormone levels drop like a barometer in a hurricane. In fact, for a significant percentage of women, menopause virtually is a two- or three-year hurricane that they profoundly wish would go away.

If this is menopause, I will gladly confess not too many men experience anything like it. No man loses ninety percent of his sex hormones in a couple of years except as the result of severe and unusual illness.

Nonetheless, men do have a menopause. It creeps in upon them stealthily, until, at last, they reach a point where they can't help noticing their muscles shrinking, their energy withering, their self-confidence crumbling, and their virility taking a tumble. By then, most men recognize reluctantly that their quality of life is shrinking like a pizza pie under sustained attack by a carload of high-school kids. Men enter a gray zone, a time they neither understand nor wish to talk about.

The male menopause is one of the most dynamic and significant events a man ever experiences, but it does not announce itself boldly. In fact, the time that elapses between the first hesitant signals of the male change of life and its full, ugly flowering can easily be ten or fifteen years.

Just as there are many symptoms of the menopause, whether male or female, so are there many causes. But the root causes are hormonal. Women's estrogen and progesterone levels fall sharply at menopause. Men's testosterone levels fall steadily decade by decade. But all men are different. There are rare males whose testosterone levels stay at or near youthful heights right into old age. And, typically, the result of such unusual elevations is . . . health.

I have measured the testosterone levels of many hundreds of men, and I have never seen an older male in excellent mental and physical health whose testosterone levels were not well within the normal range. And the healthiest, most vital individuals are always in the high normal ranges.

Does this mean that testosterone is the secret of male vitality? It is one of the secrets. But one of the most compelling and revolutionary insights in this book revolves around the relationship of the male sex to the female hormone. Testosterone does not rule the roost in lordly isolation. Estrogen can make or mar the overall functioning of the average man's body.

The fundamental metabolic fact that every doctor is aware of, though few give it much thought, is this: Estrogen is not simply a female hormone, nor is testosterone only a male hormone. The human body is far more mysterious and complex than that. Each sex has highly significant quantities of the opposite sex's major sex hormone in their bodies. Both men and women, therefore, require differing, but individually optimal, quantities of both estrogen and testosterone to activate their sexuality. That's why, in Chapter 10, we'll talk about the remarkable effect that supplemental testosterone can have on women's lives and libidos.

And, once we look at men and reflect on the role estrogen plays in their lives, we are going to find out why many otherwise good scientists have neglected testosterone replacement therapy. We are going to learn that the most common method of delivering testosterone—the testosterone injection—is radically flawed. And we are going to see why some scientists have suggested, on the basis of carefully done, competent research, that the male hormone is not as good as it's cracked up to be, not effective in treating impotence, not right for most men, not appropriate for handling the male menopause, etc. Their research was sound, but unfortunately it ignored the essential testosterone/estrogen relationship. Instead, they have studied their male patients solely on the basis of their testosterone.

When I first began treating menopausal men with the male hormone, I made the same mistake. I observed with fascination and delight the excellent improvements some men made as their testosterone levels rose. But I was sorely puzzled by the hormone's ineffectiveness in other men. It took time to understand the hormonal refinements that were at work. It took experience to realize that there is a window of optimal function for every hormone in the human body. Above all, it took measurement of estrogen levels to realize that estrogen can be as crucial as testosterone to the hormonal health of a middle-aged man. That's all that I'll say for now. Chapter 5 will spill the beans.

The Importance of the Male Menopause

It would be impossible to overemphasize the devastating effects that the menopause has on millions of men and women. Doctors know because people come and sit in our offices and tell us secrets that they wouldn't even whisper to their spouses. And once you've listened for a while to people telling you that their sex lives are crumbling, their energy is shattered, their health is growing shakier by the year—and one soon finds out that they're right on that point—one feels a very real compulsion to do something about it.

Is all this unpleasant change menopause? A whole lot of it is. Heart disease, high blood pressure, diabetes, arthritis, osteoporosis—indeed, most of the major risk factors for dying—are all intimately related to hormonal changes. To a surprising degree many of these dreadful conditions reverse themselves when a proper balancing of the hormones in the body is combined with sensible diet. As you'll see, that hormone balancing can be achieved either by various natural boosting techniques or by actual hormone replacement.

To say that the menopause is natural seems like a trivial distinction in the face of these calamities. Death is natural and inevitable, too, but many of us would like to postpone it. Moreover, I think I speak for most people when I say we would like to keep our youthful vigor throughout our lives, right up to the end. The real purpose of this book is to help make that possible.

What Happens in the Male Menopause

In men, the menopause—or andropause, as some would call it, because the male hormones are properly called androgens—is a more unpredictable process than in women. Not only because of the gradual nature of its timing but because the order in which symptoms appear vary from man to man, based on lifestyle and genetic inheritance. What many men first notice is a loss of sexual desire. However, that can simply reflect the tremendous significance that many men give to sex.

I think that more often the first sign, perhaps passing unnoticed, is a subtle downward shift in strength and energy. In some men, a depressive change in personality quite apparent to wife and friends is the first indication.

Whatever comes first, the eventual effect of the male menopause is an erosion of the underpinnings of our personal strengths, whatever they may be. Loss of athletic ability, loss of dynamic executive capabilities, loss of self-confidence, eagerness, aggressive energy—a sense of loss magnified and multiplied by the total unexpectedness of what we're undergoing. This is change, indeed. The sharp edges of youth are replaced by the well-traveled roads of habit and lethargy.

I don't know how many men have come to me and said things like, "Objectives go, confidence goes, fear comes in. I don't have the desire to do things for myself anymore. Sometimes I don't even want to go out the door in the morning. The world is gray."

Very typically, men will put these changes down to overwork, stress, the vaguely understood concept of a midlife crisis. By and large, these explanations are pap. The changes that men feel are hormonal, are real, and can be understood first and changed second. They can be measured, too.

There isn't anything all that difficult about treating the male menopause and beating it. Complicated, yes, but not difficult. And the rewards are vast. Better life, longer life, brighter, younger, more vital life. Not to mention a remarkable decrease in the risk of major diseases that jut up like rocks in the road of longevity.

This book is one piece of a hormone revolution that is happening all around us now. Laypeople and a portion of the medical profession have woken up to the fact that hormones contain the juice of youth and, without their presence in optimal quantities, vital, vigorous life is nearly impossible. I'm going to touch on the characteristics and the hormone replacement possibilities of many hormones in this book, but, by and large, this is a book about testosterone, and unashamedly so.

Testosterone is far more than just a sex hormone. Testosterone travels to every part of the human body. There are receptors for it from your brain to your toes. Testosterone is vitally involved in the making of protein, which, in turn, forms muscle. Testosterone is a key player in the manufacture of bone. Testosterone improves oxygen uptake throughout the body, vitalizing all tissues. Testosterone helps control blood sugar, helps regulate cholesterol, helps maintain a powerful immune system. Testosterone appears to help in mental concentration and improves mood. Testosterone is most likely one of the key components in protecting your brain against Alzheimer's disease.

The "male hormone" is dynamite. Don't leave home without it.

What This Book Will Show You

It's very apparent to me that if you intend to live a long, vital, healthy life then, at some point, you and your physician are going to have to address the question of your hormone levels just as seriously as physicians currently address things like blood pressure and blood sugar. You cannot retain the energy of youth—or even a small part of the energy of youth—without securing for yourself a reasonably constant supply of fairly optimal hormone levels. If you're a man, the key is usually testosterone. So, here are the things this book is going to explain:

❑ How to identify the symptoms and patterns of the male menopause
❑ What the different hormones—in particular testosterone—do for you
❑ How hormone decline is linked to the rise of late life illness and devitalization
❑ How such declines can be reversed

❑ What testosterone's specific relationship is to such critical health areas as prostate health, sexual function, bone preservation, and heart health

❑ How the many forms of the male menopause can often be treated naturally without the need for actual testosterone replacement

❑ How you can choose the best method of testosterone replacement, if you eventually require one

❑ How you can turn your health around and possibly save your life

❑ How you can enjoy the best possible sexual function in the second half of your life

❑ How to work with your doctor on replacing your testosterone at the level that's right for you; hormones are potent, powerful substances—a level that's higher than your natural norm is not at all desirable

❑ How women can get sizable health advantages from small doses of testosterone

❑ How to understand the importance of other hormonal interactions and deficiencies

❑ How to work with your doctor to create a treatment plan that's right for you

Once you've absorbed the explanations I've outlined above, you'll understand that nearly everything that tradition and observation of the people around you has taught you about the unidirectional nature of human aging is no longer completely true.

❑

After you thoroughly understand the program I've just outlined, you'll look at the male menopause differently. The human race has suffered it for a long time now, almost without recognition, certainly without giving it a name. For many men it has been, and still is, a catastrophe.

Fortunately, times change, knowledge changes, medicine changes.

CHAPTER 2:
Things That Happen to Real People

Consider two people, a man and a woman, each in their middle span of years.

A Very Common Story

Tim W. is a patient of mine, a fifty-five-year-old lawyer from central Pennsylvania, whose complaints, when I first heard them, sounded very much like "normal" aging. Tim wasn't sick, he wasn't breaking down physically or emotionally, he wasn't sexually nonfunctional.

But he wasn't well either. Tim came to me about four years ago because there were a lot of physical changes in his life, which taken one by one didn't sound particularly threatening or impressive but taken together were turning him into a different person.

He had noticed the first changes when he was around forty. He had put it down to overwork. His practice was doing well,

13

and that meant a lot of evenings and Saturday afternoons at the office. Result: sometimes he simply didn't feel like getting up in the morning. And there were other changes, too. His interest in sex had declined. A strange veneer of irritability and depression was beginning to coat the surface of his life.

Tim W. had always been athletic, but there were changes here, as well. Jogging had become a chore, not something that boosted his energy. Tennis and golf were less exhilarating.

As Tim's forties advanced, all these changes did, too. The faint shadow of depression over everything he did seemed to be growing. He was frequently tired, had difficulty concentrating on new cases, and felt little desire to initiate fresh approaches. He realized he had become more passive. His television set was a real buddy now.

And sexually he had the first fearful sense that perhaps something irreversible was happening. Tim's libido had really sunk. Occasional sexual encounters with his wife were now very occasional. When they went on vacation, things would perk up, which allowed him for a little while longer to maintain the illusion that the only problem was overwork. But Tim couldn't help noticing other, subtler sexual changes. For one thing, he no longer had early morning erections. And, when he had an orgasm, there was a radical drop-off in the volume of ejaculate. Moreover, at ejaculation the intensity of pleasure had declined. He didn't think much about sex at all now, and he began to suspect his body was telling him something.

Tim is exactly the sort of person to whom ten years ago I would have said, "Some changes you have to expect when you're over fifty. We all get older, and it certainly doesn't sound like there's anything serious here for you to worry about."

Nothing serious except the whole quality of his life, his sense of self-esteem, perhaps his marriage, and, in the long run, probably his health. Since traditional medical dogma was that there was no male menopause, I certainly hadn't known any better. By the time Tim came to see me, I was smart enough to suggest we measure his testosterone levels. Tim's testosterone was 190 nanograms per deciliter (ng/dl), a good deal less than half what one would expect in a man his age and perhaps a quarter of the average in young men. (Normal range is defined as between 350 and 1000 ng/dl.) Once I looked at this number, I was not surprised that Tim was tired, irritable, sexually quiescent, and off his game, in every sense.

Every symptom I've described so far rapidly reversed itself with replacement doses of testosterone. Tim's wife found a reinvigorated romantic partner, his golfing buddies at the country club discovered—perhaps to their dismay—that old Tim was suddenly driving the ball twenty yards further than he used to, and Tim himself realized that his life was not winding down, that he was not stuck in the mud, that he was himself again— morning erections and career motivation both restored. He now had energy that he hadn't seen since his thirties.

This may be the simplest story that I'll tell you in this book. Tim can stand in for many men. I could easily go into my records and find fifty Tims. Not sick, not well—men who were simply wondering what in the dickens had happened to the man they used to know.

Janice D.—Coming Alive Again

Janice D. was fifty-seven and still very much in love with life. Enthusiastic, creative, an artist, she has always been prone to point out that half-empty glasses are half full. She was adept at adapting. But she was noticing changes. Less energy, problems with bladder leakage, loss of muscular strength. It was getting harder to pick up her grandchildren. They hadn't gotten that much bigger in just the past year!

And then there was a vast vacancy in her life that wasn't new. It had started twenty years ago, when she was suddenly diagnosed with endometrial and uterine cancer and had to have a hysterectomy, followed by radiation. The results were sexually devastating. Janice lost all sexual urges, and, in any event, the skin of her vagina was so thin, dry, and fragile that, on the rare occasions when she had intercourse with her husband, pain was the only possible sensory experience for her.

Janice had adapted (and somehow her husband had, too). Being a very positive person, she was just glad to be alive. For a time she was put on estrogen, but it made her feel depressed. A doctor put her on methyl testosterone at one point, but it did not help much. Very soon, she was taken off it.

Janice went on through the next two decades aware that a whole dimension of being alive was missing for her but enjoying most other aspects of her life. She came to see me in the summer of 1996. Loss of strength, lower energy, and bladder leakage were bothering her. She didn't expect any change in her sexual status.

I switched her to estradiol, a natural form of estrogen identical to her own normal estrogen, then gave her small amounts of pure testosterone, in a cream that would be absorbed directly into the bloodstream. Some of the cream was to be applied to the vulvar area, where natural testosterone receptors activate the normal sexual responses. I also had her use it in a vaginal cream to strengthen muscles that control the bladder. The muscles in that portion of women's bodies are packed with testosterone receptors. Janice saw changes very quickly:

> *In just a few weeks I saw the hormones I was taking creating a new me. I had much greater and more constant energy throughout the day. I felt physically stronger. But the most startling change was sexual. I*

woke up. I began to feel desire again. I felt alive. My husband was amazed. And it became physically possible to have intercourse again. Now my vagina is pink and moist and strong. I've plumped out down there.

I don't know why more women don't know about testosterone. Sometimes I see women in the supermarket who I think look and feel the way I did before. I'd like to tell them that this so-called male hormone has made me feel more womanly than I've ever felt before.

What Janice has told me repeatedly is that now she feels fully alive. All the other improvements in her health and energy, which she originally came to see me about, are just a bonus.

One Study

As you've just seen, replacing depleted levels of testosterone can significantly alter the quality of men's and women's lives. I've seen this so many times—hundreds of times—that I'm no longer particularly surprised when it happens. I watch people in their forties, fifties, and sixties emerging out of the gray zone like a butterfly out of its chrysalis.

I suppose, observing these changes, that you would assume medicine was just now catching wind of what testosterone can do. You would expect many studies to have been done in recent years (and they have been), and you would think regretfully about how nice it would have been if anyone had thought to test for the health-restoring capacities of the male hormone a long time ago, so that this medical breakthrough could have started much earlier.

As a matter of fact, the first clear evidence for testosterone's potent effect in aging males was presented more than fifty years ago. This research by Dr. Carl Heller and Dr. Gordon Myers was published in the Journal of the American Medical Association.[1] It was a well-designed study that sought to determine whether testosterone levels were in any way related to some of the typical midlife changes in men. Could it be that there was a male menopause, or a "climacteric," as it was referred to then?

The researchers took thirty-eight men who had a wide variety of midlife symptoms (summarized in Table 1) and measured their hormonal status. They also measured the levels of twenty-five healthy, nonsymptomatic men ranging in age from twenty-two to ninety-eight. All the healthy controls had normal sexual function (yes, even the ninety-eight-year-old!), normal testicular function, and, as they soon discovered, normal testosterone levels.

In the thirty-eight men with midlife health problems, the researchers got an interesting result. Not all of them had testosterone deficiency—as we've said, aging is a combination of many factors and rates of testosterone decline vary widely from man to man. But twenty-three of the thirty-eight did.

The doctors decided to find out what would happen if all these men were put on testosterone. They gave injections of testosterone propionate, 25 milligrams (mg) five times weekly, for two to four weeks to everyone. The twenty-five healthy high-testosterone men showed no significant change in health, energy, or mood. The fifteen men who combined sexual dysfunction with normal testosterone levels also showed no change. But the twenty men remaining in the study (three had dropped out), who not only had symptoms of the midlife gray zone but who had low testosterone levels as well, began to change.

By the second week, definite improvements were noted in all twenty. By the end of the third week, nearly all symptoms had been "cured" in seventeen out of the twenty men. Three of the men still had depression or other disorders of mood, and it was

Table 1: *Symptoms Cited By Heller and Myers*

Psychic:	**Constitutional:**
nervousness	weakness
irritability	fatigue
insomnia	muscle pains
depression	nausea and vomiting
antisocial tendencies	constipation
crying spells	weight loss
suicidal tendencies	
inability to concentrate	**Urinary:**
	decreased force
Vasomotor:	frequency
hot flashes	hesitancy
chilliness	
sweating	
palpitation	**Sexual:**
increased pulse rate	diminution of libido
headache	decreased erections

concluded that in their cases there were complicating psychological factors. Sexual potency returned to normal in eighteen of the twenty men. In the two men remaining, the dosage was then doubled, and these men, too, found that their sexual vigor was largely restored.

Testosterone was later withheld from some of the twenty men and their symptoms, including lack of sexual potency, returned.

Doctors Heller and Myers concluded that what they referred to as the male climacteric did exist and that it was possible to diagnose it and to treat it with testosterone. They speculated that it was a rare disorder, but, as you'll see, this was one area in which their conclusions have not stood the test of time. With today's refinements in hormone testing, relative hormonal deficiency and hormonal imbalances are common.

The absence of reaction to their study is puzzling. The popular medical writer, Paul de Kruif, had publicized the notion of testosterone therapy for men in an article in *Reader's Digest* that year and was soon to write a book on the subject. Dutch doctors had created a synthetic form of testosterone in 1935, so administration of the hormone was not an obstacle. Nonetheless, a vast silence descended over the field.

Burying the Male Menopause

The silence is about to end. As you'll soon see in detail, testosterone has the capacity to drastically alter the course of aging, radically improve the quality of life, and change both the risk of experiencing many aging diseases in the middle and later years and the course of treatment, if and when they occur. In conjunction with the other hormones, it is capable of changing the entire second half of life.

But, just like the other hormones, its effectiveness is limited to individuals who are out of balance or declining away from youthful healthy levels. Eventually, that means most of us. For you and for every other person who reads this book, the rate at which you reach relative depletion will be individualized and largely unpredictable. It is possible, however, to come to a shrewd judgement as to just where you are by looking at the composite of symptoms that you already have and by doing specific lab tests. The next chapter is dedicated to showing you how you can conduct a self-analysis, a self-testing that will reveal much. Are you in the gray zone of the male menopause? Let's find out.

CHAPTER 3:

Are You in the Gray Zone Yet?

We all age. Most of us observe this process unethusiastically and would slow it if we could. In this book I want to make it possible for you to determine how far along you are in aging. Once you have that information, you'll be better prepared to decide what you want to do about it. You might even decide to reverse the process.

Most likely you think this sounds bizarre. Reverse aging? Surely it's just as easy to tell the sun to stand still.

Not really. It's certainly true that in the past nothing could be done about aging. You knew then that whatever way you felt at the present time, you were certainly going to feel a little older in a year or two. The process was irreversible, steady, and downhill.

This simply isn't true any longer. A carefully planned program of diet, exercise, and hormonal boosting or replacement can make you feel younger a year or two from now than you do today. I've seen it happen faster than that. And the lucky people who experienced these changes weren't just younger in their own minds. Their outward appearance, their metabolic functioning as measured by lab tests, their everyday standard of behavior—energy, attitude, drive—were all testimony to the fact that, for a while at least, they would enjoy the very special pleasure of spitting in the face of the calendar.

Before we consider whether you, too, can objectively speaking make yourself feel younger, it makes good sense to establish a personal baseline. There are clusters of significant symptoms in such areas as brain function, sex function, general metabolic condition, and musculoskeletal wellness that go a long way toward determining how far you've traveled from the blithe days of your youth.

I want you to look at the symptoms outlined below and, to the best of your knowledge, decide whether you've seen noticeable or significant declines in any of these areas of function in the years since you turned thirty-five. It is, of course, perfectly normal to see a certain amount of decline in some aspects of physical function. Nobody's perfect; we all age, and, certainly, not many people are as athletic at fifty-five as they were at thirty-five. In fact, at the high end of functionality, nobody is.

Nonetheless, if you find yourself racking up too many moderate or major decreases in function, that probably indicates you're aging faster than you need to, and it may well reflect hormonal decline.

So please make an honest effort, examine your physiological conscience, and let's see what answers you come up with.

Sex Function

Decrease in spontaneous early morning erections
❑ Rare   ❑ Moderate   ❑ Frequent

Decreased libido or desire for sex
❑ Rare   ❑ Moderate   ❑ Frequent

Decrease in fullness of erections
❑ Rare   ❑ Moderate   ❑ Frequent

Decrease in volume of ejaculate or semen
❑ Rare   ❑ Moderate   ❑ Frequent

Decrease in strength of climax or force of muscular pulsations
❑ Rare   ❑ Moderate   ❑ Frequent

Difficulty in maintaining full erection
❑ Rare   ❑ Moderate   ❑ Frequent

Difficulty in starting erection—or no erection
❑ Rare   ❑ Moderate   ❑ Frequent

Mental Functions

Spells of mental fatigue or inability to concentrate; feeling burned out
❑ Rare   ❑ Moderate   ❑ Frequent

Tiredness or sleepiness in the afternoon or early evening
❑ Rare   ❑ Moderate   ❑ Frequent

Decrease in mental sharpness, attention, wit
❑ Rare   ❑ Moderate   ❑ Frequent

Change in creativity or spontaneous new ideas
❑ Rare   ❑ Moderate   ❑ Frequent

Decrease in initiative or desire to start new projects
❏ Rare   ❏ Moderate   ❏ Frequent

Decreased interest in past hobbies or new work-related activities
❏ Rare   ❏ Moderate   ❏ Frequent

Decrease in competitiveness
❏ Rare   ❏ Moderate   ❏ Frequent

Change in memory function; increased forgetfulness
❏ Rare   ❏ Moderate   ❏ Frequent

Feeling of depression; a sense that work, marriage, or recreational activities have lost significance
❏ Rare   ❏ Moderate   ❏ Frequent

Musculoskeletal Condition

"Sore-body syndrome"—aches, joint and muscle pains
❏ Rare   ❏ Moderate   ❏ Frequent

Decline in flexibility and mobility; increased stiffness
❏ Rare   ❏ Moderate   ❏ Frequent

Decrease in muscle size, tone, strength
❏ Rare   ❏ Moderate   ❏ Frequent

Decrease in physical stamina
❏ Rare   ❏ Moderate   ❏ Frequent

Decrease in athletic performance
❏ Rare   ❏ Moderate   ❏ Frequent

Back pain; neck pain
❏ Rare   ❏ Moderate   ❏ Frequent

Tendency to pull muscles or get leg cramps
❏ Rare   ❏ Moderate   ❏ Frequent

Development of osteoporosis or inflammatory arthritis (rheumatoid arthritis)
❑ Rare   ❑ Moderate   ❑ Frequent

Metabolic or Physical/Disease Problems

Increase in total cholesterol or triglycerides
❑ Rare   ❑ Moderate   ❑ Frequent

Decrease in HDL cholesterol
❑ Rare   ❑ Moderate   ❑ Frequent

Rise in blood sugar level or diabetes onset
❑ Rare   ❑ Moderate   ❑ Frequent

Rise in blood pressure/diagnosis of hypertension
❑ Rare   ❑ Moderate   ❑ Frequent

Unexplained weight gain, particularly in the midsection; "beer belly" (waist-to-hip ratio)
❑ Rare   ❑ Moderate   ❑ Frequent

Increased fat distribution in breast area or hips
❑ Rare   ❑ Moderate   ❑ Frequent

Development of chest pain, or diagnosis of heart disease or blockage in arteries
❑ Rare   ❑ Moderate   ❑ Frequent

Shortness of breath with activities; worsening of asthma or emphysema
❑ Rare   ❑ Moderate   ❑ Frequent

Lightheadedness, dizzy spells, or ringing of the ears; new onset of headaches
❑ Rare   ❑ Moderate   ❑ Frequent

Poor circulation in legs, swelling of ankles, development of varicose veins or hemorrhoids
❏ Rare   ❏ Moderate   ❏ Frequent

Changes in visual acuity, focus reading fine print
❏ Rare   ❏ Moderate   ❏ Frequent

For you, the purpose of this quiz has been to get you thinking about how far you've advanced into the gray zone of middle age. Many of these apparently unconnected symptoms are not so unconnected after all, but actually correspond remarkably well with the expected results of hormonal deprivation. For instance, lower levels of testosterone and estrogen have serious deleterious effects on the proper functioning of the brain, resulting in a decrease in mental sharpness. This means that these hormones, whose functions would appear to be limited since we refer to them as "sex" hormones, turn out to also be brain hormones. And, as you'll soon see, testosterone and estrogen are also muscle hormones and bone hormones, skin hormones and energy hormones, mood hormones and urinary tract hormones. So, when we refer to them as sex hormones, important as sexual functions are, we are certainly demonstrating the deceptive possibilities of language.

At the same time, it's clear that not all aging is hormonal. There are certain standard patterns of aging decline that seem to occur in everyone. There is, for instance, a decline in the focusability of the eyes, which appears to be universal. There is a steady loss of lung function. There is a decline in kidney function. But even here one wonders whether some part of this seemingly universal and irreversible decline is not hormonal. Studies, both in animals and people, have shown that the shrinking of major organs such as the liver and kidney, which is so characteristic of aging, can be partly reversed by the adminis-

tration of human growth hormone. After many months of hormone replacement, the organs regenerate, becoming larger and
more resilient.

Certainly there are parts of aging that are not hormonal, but
it's not always easy to say which parts. In the next chapter, I'll
describe the functioning of testosterone and the other endocrine
hormones, and you'll see what I mean.

CHAPTER 4:

The Hormone Universe

The patient, a man in his late sixties, had retired ten years before from the teamsters. Once he had been a fairly big man, but his clothes now seemed to hang loosely and a trifle incongruously on a body that was still getting used to its own frailty. Sam W. wanted to know why his muscles had shrunk, his gait grown halting, why his energy was entirely a thing of the past. And I could honestly tell him that while some of this was the weight of his years, most of it was plain hormone deficiency. I only had to look at his testosterone level of 175 ng/dl to know that the seventy-year-old Sam I intended to help create would be remarkably more vigorous than the sixty-nine-year-old Sam I saw in front of me now.

When I looked at Sam's levels of DHEA and human growth hormone, I was equally impressed with how low they were and with how big a difference replacing those missing hormones was going to make.

Praise for the Hormone Empire

As we go from youth to age and health to disease, hormonal changes are the single most important transforming factor. If you would like to stay healthy far into old age, possessed of energy and vitality, nothing you do can match in significance retaining youthful levels of your major hormones. By replacing those hormones when necessary, you can gain a reprieve of sentence from aging.

The fact that you were once bursting with vitality, ready to leap fences, climb mountains, and conquer worlds was not an accident of youth. It *was* youth, which is largely an expression of hormonal strength. The rare people who astonish the world with their activities in their seventies and eighties would astonish the lab technicians if anybody took their hormone levels. Hormones are the fuel of youth. They fight infection and heal injury, cause you to grow, fine-tune the way you deal with stress, control your inner heating apparatus, permit and encourage a good night's sleep, balance the levels of minerals in your body, adjust the burning of fuel for energy, and, of course, underlie your sex drive.

Let's briefly look at all the major endocrine hormones. These are the hormones that are secreted directly into your bloodstream from glands called the endocrine glands. From there they get carried to other organs and tissues throughout your body.

Suppose you're walking across the street when suddenly a runaway truck comes roaring your way. You leap across the distance separating you from the sidewalk, and it misses you by inches. You notice that you're trembling, that your heart is pounding, that your physical reaction is entirely out of proportion to the physical effort you just made. In fact, you're dealing with an adrenaline surge, which the body was able to send forth in the time it took you to save your life.

Adrenaline is simply one of the most spectacular of this wildly powerful and efficient team of natural substances. Here are the hormones we're going to glance at before we go back to focusing on testosterone:

- ❑ estrogen
- ❑ progesterone
- ❑ insulin
- ❑ adrenaline
- ❑ DHEA (dehydroepiandrosterone)
- ❑ thyroid hormone
- ❑ melatonin
- ❑ human growth hormone
- ❑ pituitary hormones
- ❑ hypothalamic hormones

Pertaining to the Female

Many of the physical characteristics of femininity are, of course, made possible by estrogen, the dominant hormone in the ovaries. Like testosterone it is an anabolic steroid, though its anabolic (muscle-building) effect is significantly weaker. Its effect on physical shape, on fat deposits around hips and breasts and thighs, is well known. It's also a powerful protector of bone, a guardian of female cardiovascular health, a promoter of thick, smooth skin, and, naturally, a crucial component in the proper functioning of the female sex organs. Chapter 5 will offer a more exhaustive discussion of this amazing hormone.

The other major female hormone, progesterone, also produced primarily in the ovaries, causes the lining of the uterus to thicken in preparation for pregnancy, and, when pregnancy occurs, is essential for normal functioning and the healthy development of the baby. At the end of pregnancy, a fall in the level of progesterone helps initiate labor. These two hormones are, of course, the basic team in most of the hormone replacement therapies currently being done on postmenopausal women. Originally estrogen was replaced alone, but doctors discovered this increased the risk of uterine cancer and so progesterone was added. There also appear to be other benefits from progesterone replacement, and I'll explain them in Chapter 10.

Not Just for Diabetics

Proceeding upwards in this quick tour of the endocrine glands, we come to the pancreas, the source of insulin, the hormone that Type I diabetics cannot produce and must replace daily to survive. Insulin is released whenever we eat and facilitates the transport of blood sugar (glucose) into our cells for fuel. Some of the glucose gets stored in the liver and muscles as glycogen, a complex carbohydrate that the body can call upon to meet energy needs. If insulin is not doing its job properly, then the excess glucose is more easily stored as fat and the breakdown of fat for energy is also impaired.

Insulin frequently becomes a hormonal problem as we get older; the body uses it less efficiently and the resulting condition, called insulin resistance, is associated with increased obesity, high blood pressure, and cardiovascular risk. Careful diet and exercise can minimize the problem, and, as we'll see, testosterone has a role to play as well.

Mighty Powerful Little Organs

The next stage in our upward progression toward the brain is the adrenals, two small but critical glands that sit atop the kidneys. In their center (the medulla), the adrenals produce adrenaline, our fight-or-flight emergency action hormone. Adrenaline ignites a high-speed burnoff of the glycogen we previously mentioned. This is converted more or less instantaneously to glucose, fueling the energy for action.

On the outer layer (the cortex) of the adrenals, a major hormone, DHEA (dehydroepiandrosterone) is manufactured from cholesterol. Nearly every cell in the body has receptor sites for this unique hormone, but its exact purpose is only dimly understood.

There are three things we definitely do know about DHEA. First, that it declines steadily in the human body after early adulthood. Second, that men and women who are middle-aged or older generally feel marked improvements in well-being when they take replacement doses of DHEA. Third, that DHEA can be converted to many other hormones in the body, including testosterone and estrogen.

The Heat Hormone

Just beneath the voice box at the front of the throat is a little butterfly shaped gland called the thyroid. This gland regulates our metabolism by controlling the production of energy in our cells. The fuel from food and stored fat combines with oxygen in our cells. This produces the chemical energy that powers all the functions of our body from movement to thought. The thyroid hormone, thyroxin, is the regulator of this process and the controller of our body heat and rate of cellular activity.

Most of us will never have a thyroid problem and will never need to replace the thyroid hormone. However, approximately 20 percent of people over sixty—women more commonly than men—do have such problems. Hypothyroidism—low thyroid— is the more common disease state. Symptoms of deficiency include fatigue, chilliness, cold hands and feet, numbness and weakness in the hands, constipation, poor memory, dull hair, and dry skin. Overproduction of thyroid hormone causes fatigue, anxiety, weight loss, and racing heart.

Modern medicine can normalize the thyroid, if the condition is properly diagnosed.

The Hormones as a Team

I know this wide spectrum of important hormones sounds fairly complicated. You might well wonder how the body can sort out their overlapping functions and cause them to work together.

By and large, the body does a superlative job. Your metabolism in tune, functioning well, is like a symphony orchestra with all the musicians playing harmoniously together, joined in one happy purpose.

Scientists now believe that the orchestra conductor, the force responsible for controlling the instruments and forging unity out of what could easily be chaos, is the pituitary gland and its related control center, the hypothalamus. The pituitary, a small organ at the base of your brain, is hidden and protected in the middle of the head. Weighing in at less than a gram (one-fortieth of an ounce), it is connected by a thin stalk to the hypothalamus, which is the lowermost part of the brain itself. The two glands are so closely interconnected that, for practical purposes, they can hardly be thought of separately.

These master glands are the overlords of your hormone empire. They send hormonal messengers to the other glands, bearing precise directions for appropriate secretions of all the hormones we've been talking about. Actually, the pituitary sends the messengers, and the hypothalamus tells it what to send. For instance, by means of a hormone called ACTH (adrenal cortical stimulating hormone), the pituitary governs the output of specific adrenal cortical hormones by the adrenal gland. In a similar fashion, it directs the production of the sex hormones through pituitary controlling hormones called gonadotrophins (-*trophic* means *to stimulate the growth of*). All the other endocrine glands we've discussed also receive peremptory messages from the control team in the brain.

If, as a result of these communications, the quantities of hormones and the timing of their release are ideally suited to your needs then the result will be optimal physical and mental performance. The orchestra is playing your tune. You know it, you feel it throughout the course of every restful night and energetic day. You're really living.

In contrast to this happy picture, illness or aging may eventually appear. Then, the music loses harmony. A wrong note is struck first here, and then there, and soon, it sometimes seems, almost everywhere. Aging is a breakdown in the perfect music of youth. Something has changed. The stresses of life have upset the woodwinds, or some genetic inheritance slowly working its way to the surface has thrown the horns into disorder. Perhaps some viral or bacterial onslaught has literally damaged the quality of the instruments.

Most commonly, however—even in the absence of disease—the endocrine glands lose the capacity to manufacture their hormones in the quantities necessary for playing the beautiful music of youth. And when the balance and quantity of your hormones is not ideal, your body begins striking dreadfully sour notes. This is basic medicine, though often overlooked.

It's also possible—as we'll see in a moment—for the control glands, the hypothalamus and the pituitary, to lose their capacity to send the proper instructions. For most of our hormone systems, this seems to be less common than a failing productive capacity. That may not be true, however, in the case of testosterone.

Before we proceed to testosterone, let's not forget to mention one other hormone that shares many characteristics with it. I'm referring to human growth hormone (HGH), an extremely important product of the pituitary gland. Human growth hormone is necessary for the normal growth of children and, until HGH replacement became possible, children who were deficient in it reached maturity as dwarfs. Because of its name and its known function in young people, it was assumed that HGH was not particularly important in adults. We now know that HGH is one of the body's main maintenance and repair hormones and that the sizable loss of it that occurs as we age can have serious effects on health, leading— among many other things—to weakness, frailty, and diminished immune function. In the last few years, more and more people have been taking HGH as an anti-aging replacement medicine, and the results have frequently been impressive. I'll discuss this powerful (and expensive) hormone at greater length in Chapter 11.

Filling Out the Testosterone Picture

Testosterone is an anabolic steroid, which means not only that it possesses a unique chemical structure but that it has the capacity to promote the formation of bone and muscle in the body. Testosterone is also referred to as an androgen, which means "male producing." And, certainly, the hormone is an essential component of maleness.

In fact, there's a sense in which it is testosterone that makes men male. You see, all fetuses start out anatomically female. If, however, the sperm that reached the egg carried a Y chromosome, then, sometime in the second month after conception, the male chromosome will cause the embryo's newly developing genital ridge to secrete testosterone. As a result, the male sexual organs will begin to form.

Those organs are well equipped to produce testosterone. Specialized cells in the testicles called Leydig cells become the male's main factory for testosterone production and eventually form approximately 20 percent of the total testicular mass.

In adult males approximately 90 to 95 percent of testosterone is produced in the testicles by the Leydig cells, and the remainder is secreted as yet another product of the adrenals, those small, spectacularly potent glands we discussed a few pages back.

In women, approximately half the testosterone produced comes from the ovaries and about half from the adrenal glands. Some is also created elsewhere in the body by conversion from the adrenal hormone, DHEA. During the menstrual years, these various sources of the male hormone give the average woman a level about one-tenth as high as that of the average man. But, by her mid-thirties, a woman's adrenal production begins to fall off dramatically, although sometimes not right away. That's because, as the ovaries begin to fail, the body sends surges of gonadotrophins to promote estrogen production. Frequently, all they can manage to do is increase testosterone, an estrogen precursor. Thus, there may be a temporary rise in the male hormone. If, at that point, a woman goes on estrogen replacement, however, testosterone will quickly fall. This is yet another reason why a modest replacement dose of testosterone as an accompaniment to estrogen replacement makes very good sense for menopausal women.

Since I'll be discussing testosterone in the female in Chapter 10, let's concentrate on the changes that occur in the male.

First, There's Puberty

Throughout childhood the male is producing rather small amounts of testosterone, and his Leydig cells are relatively quiescent. Then, at around thirteen years of age, puberty strikes. The control panel in the brain has sent signals to the testes to pour out the testosterone. Teenage girls receive similar instructions for estrogen (and, secondarily, for testosterone). All the changes we're familar with begin to occur. In teenage boys the sexual organs enlarge, pubic and axillary hair grows, the voice deepens due to the thickening of the vocal cords, there is a thickening and darkening of the skin, an enlargement of the skeletal structure, a considerable increase in musclature, and, of course, the onset of sexual sensations and desires. There's nothing subtle about testosterone at puberty. This is a blowtorch of a hormone.

Teenage girls have their own quite apparent changes. The result, as we've all noticed, is that boys and girls lose the rather androgynous appearance of children and are suddenly transformed into two distinctly different body types.

By their late teens, males are at their lifetime high levels of testosterone, typically 800 to 1200 ng/dl when blood testing is done. Those levels usually stay fairly constant for the next ten to twenty years. Then they begin to decline, according to one study, at an average rate of 1 percent a year for total testosterone and 1.2 percent a year for the very important free testosterone. That, however, is no more than a statistical average. Male testosterone decline is highly variable and dependant on many interlocking individual factors. Some men are in the andropause by the time they're forty and measure only 200 to 300 ng/dl when tested. Other men are still at 800 ng/dl at seventy.

Why does testosterone decline? The rest of this chapter will give the first part of that answer; the next chapter, the surprising last part.

Testosterone in Men: Two Ways to Fall

We don't actually know *why* testosterone declines, but we certainly know *how* it declines. There are two commonly recognized endocrine disorders that can cause a man to have low blood levels of testosterone.[1] We're going to discuss these right now, but, in the next chapter, we'll consider a third type of testosterone disorder that doesn't necessarily involve declining levels of the hormone and whose significance has consequently been wildly underrated. This is what you'll come to know as metabolic andropause, and it may be even more important than a straightforward testosterone deficiency.

The two well-recognized types of deficiency are classically known as primary and secondary hypogonadism—hypogonadism is simply a term referring to underactivity of the sexual organs or gonads. (*Hypo-* is a term in medicine that always means *low*, just as *hyper-* means *high*—therefore, hypogonadal means low gonadal function.) Hypogonadic men are producing smaller than normal amounts of testosterone in their testicles resulting in deficient blood levels of the hormone. This can be happening because the testicular Leydig cells have lost the capacity to secrete the hormone at youthful levels (primary hypogonadism). Alternatively, the Leydig cell capacity may be unimpaired, but the control glands in the brain are not asking them to use that capacity. The pituitary ought to be dispatching hormonal messengers with stern demands for more testosterone. For some reason these peremptory requests are not being sent often enough or hard enough. That's secondary hypogonadism.

Let's consider how the system works and what goes wrong when it goes awry.

Isn't Anyone in Charge Here?

To regulate any aspect of the body's functioning, the brain has to know what's going on. The hypothalamus is the knowledgeable portion of the hypothalamus/pituitary team. It has sensors that detect circulating blood levels of the many specific hormones that the pituitary controls. Acting like a rheostat, it sends messages to the pituitary telling it to turn production by the lower endocrine centers up or down as needed. The system is extremely clever, and, in young people, it almost invariably hums along as smoothly as a high-quality Swiss timepiece.

In the case of testosterone, when the hypothalamus detects that levels are not as high as they ought to be, it sends brief bursts of a hormone called GnRH (gonadotrophin-releasing hormone) to the pituitary. This stimulates the pituitary to secrete LH (lutenizing hormone) and FSH (follicle-stimulating hormone) at about hourly intervals.

LH and FSH are referred to collectively as the gonadotrophins, meaning hormones that exert an influence on the sex glands. These gonadotrophins stimulate the Leydig cells in the testicles to manufacture testosterone. The whole production process is regulated by what scientists call a feedback system. This means that the hypothalamus monitors the levels of testosterone in the blood, and, if those levels rise too high, the

Table 2: *Causes of Hypogonadism*

Primary:	Secondary:
hemochromotosis	pituitary or hypothalamic tumor
AIDs	granulomatous disease
cancer	infarction
chronic disease	trauma
rheumatoid arthritis	vascular defects
renal failure	hyperprolactinemia
cirrhosis of the liver	nutritional deficiency or starvation
chronic obstructive pulmonary disease	massive obesity
	glucocorticoid drugs
drugs (cancer chemotherapy or immunosuppressants)	Kallman's syndrome
radiation	isolated deficiency of luteinizing hormone or follicle-stimulating hormone
alcohol	genetic disorder:
	Prader-Willi syndrome
	Laurence-Moon-Biedi syndrome
	delayed puberty

hypothalamus down-regulates its signals to the pituitary. The pituitary then slows its secretions of gonadotrophins and less testosterone is produced for a while, until finally the hypothalamus decides the system needs upregulating.

Tired Gland

So, what has happened to this economical and efficient system when a man's testosterone levels are too low? In the case of primary hypogonadism, the problem is in the testicles themselves. The Leydig cells have lost a measure of their natural capacity to secrete the hormone. When this occurs, the hypothalamus notices that not enough testosterone is being produced and tells the pituitary to pump out more LH and FSH to stimulate the Leydig cells. But this stimulation is to no avail. Generally speaking, if blood tests are done in such a situation, it will be found that levels of the gonadotrophins are unusually high, indicating an ongoing effort by the pituitary and the hypothalamus to stimulate activity. To an endocrinologist, high gonadotrophins combined with low testosterone spell out classical testicular failure.

Secondary hypogonadism is a condition in which disorders of the hypothalamus or the pituitary disorders cripple their secretion of the gonadotrophins. In the relative (or complete) absence of these hormonal messengers, the testicles lower (or halt) their production of testosterone even though the still healthy and efficient Leydig cells would be perfectly capable of producing it if proper stimulation were provided.

In my experience, secondary hypogonadism is the more common cause of testosterone deficiency in middle-aged men. Often it's not clear what the source of this defect in the hormonal system is. Some form of vascular damage may interrupt the pathways leading from the hypothalamus to the pituitary. Severe viral infections or autoimmune disease may cause damage to these central nervous system endocrine glands. There may be not-yet-discovered drug interactions that cause damage and, in some cases, nutritional deficiencies may be implicated.

The attractive thing about secondary hypogonadism is that when it occurs it is usually treatable. There is a hormone called chorionic gonadotrophin (CG) that is very similar in molecular function to LH, which we will discuss in more detail in Chapter 13. Generally speaking, CG is entirely effective at jump-starting the quiescent testes.

Teddy B., who came to see me because, in his words, "I'm feeling crappy," is a good illustration of what occurs. Teddy is a hard-working fifty-two-year-old businessman who wondered where his energy went. I did lab tests and discovered that his testosterone was 272 ng/dl—off the scales by any standard. His levels of FSH and LH were low, which suggested that the problem lay with his central control panel. Requests for more testosterone simply weren't being sent down.

I tried him on chorionic gonadotrophin, and one month later his testosterone was 1114 ng/dl, which is a little bit off the scales at the high end. Teddy's fatigue was going away in a rush, but he did feel slightly irritable with almost an excess of manic energy. We adjusted his dose down from three times a week to twice, his testosterone went down into the 800s, and Teddy felt just fine, just like his old, high-energy self. It was a perfect case of secondary hypogonadism, hormonally adjusted.

Such successes are exciting, but it has been my experience that the most significant form of male menopause is not caused by a deficiency of testosterone (whether primary or secondary) but by a significantly more complicated form of hormone disorder. Let's turn to the next chapter and find out about it.

CHAPTER 5:

Estrogen—The Culprit

Many men who can boast normal levels of testosterone nonetheless exhibit characteristic symptoms of the male menopause. They're suffering from the third form of andropause that I promised to talk about at the end of the last chapter. For these men, too, middle-age strikes hard. They find their energy diminishing and their sexual life faltering. Yet their testosterone has not fallen through the floor.

Those among their doctors who have some comprehension of what might be happening to them shake their heads in puzzlement and say, "See, hormones aren't so important after all." The truth is quite the opposite. Hormones are amazingly important all the time and in everyone. But in this situation, the hormonal imbalance is not related to testosterone. It is in the level of estrogen, the female hormone, that the trouble lies.

Because the relationship I'm about to explain is poorly understood, this chapter is likely to be the most significant and will certainly be the most unexpected in this book. You must understand the slightly technical metabolic processes covered in this chapter or you won't really appreciate why the male menopause is such a dominating factor in the lives of the majority of men who've reached their middle years. So listen carefully while I explain the changes in male and female hormones alike that dominate so much of the male life cycle—that make the male menopause happen!

We will find that many researchers have neglected estrogen's role in males, much as they have neglected testosterone's role in females. This is not very good science. In the bodies of both men and women, the balance of these two hormones is critical. By neglecting the effects of estrogen in males, scientists have found themselves at a loss to explain the failure of testosterone replacement therapy in many men who seem ideally suited to it. Observing these failures, all too many physicians have fallen back on the assumption that testosterone is not related in any very significant way to male midlife changes. Consequently, it could not very well be part of the solution a man should be seeking to find.

Impotence—by no means an inevitable result of the male menopause but certainly a threatening one—is an intriguing example of these misperceptions. Physicians who specialize in this area will generally quote standard studies claiming that only about 5 percent of impotent men can be effectively treated with testosterone. My own experiences have taught me that the number is closer to 60 to 80 percent, though, in a majority of cases, the causes are multifactorial. The doctors who contend otherwise are, of course, sincere—they simply haven't recognized the significance of estrogen in the potency equation.

It's time to introduce you to the world of "metabolic" andropause.

Estrogen, the Forgotten Side of Masculinity

Women react with surprise when they learn the female body contains its own natural supply of testosterone. Men are equally unprepared for the news that estrogen is part of them, a perfectly normal aspect of their hormonal makeup. The male body actually manufactures its own supply of the female hormone. Where does it get it? It makes it out of that most masculine of all substances, testosterone. An enzyme called aromatase is widely present in the body and converts a certain portion of the male hormone into the female. The human body is expert at such processes, and, incidentally, the conversion itself is not such a big trick. The two hormones are chemically quite similar!

I believe that men's bodies would not have a process for making estrogen if it were useless to them. Therefore, this conversion process is actually necessary for the healthy functioning of estrogen-sensitive tissues in a man's body. As you'll see in the chapter on growth hormone, where we discuss mental function, it is likely that estrogen is powerfully beneficial to the male brain. It is certainly important in influencing certain natural sexual functions through its effects on brain chemistry. Too little estrogen will neuter a man just as effectively as too little testosterone. In point of fact, this only happens in the case of rather rare endocrine disorders. The very areas of the male brain that control sexual function are plentifully supplied with the aromatase enzyme and thus have no difficulty converting testosterone to estrogen for its special purposes in those specific locations.

When it comes to estrogen, the window of optimum effectiveness in the male body is very small. Estrogen converted by aromatase can actually unlock or displace testosterone at its various cellular receptor sites. Consequently, too much estrogen will switch off activities. In some cases, it may well be meant to. The body depends on various on/off switches to regulate the force of its actions. Since testosterone is a powerful stimulant and energizer, estrogen may very logically be a complementary off switch. The briefest consideration of sexual desire in young males, for instance, might well imply the necessity of an off switch to turn down the male libido, since unbridled sexual energy can be totally disruptive to life.

Estrogen, when it goes above its normal "window," may supply that switch even though we know that simultaneously it is making sexuality possible in certain areas of the brain. If this theory of estrogen's use is correct, then, in young people, the control it exercises can only be beneficial. In older men, however, estrogen's rise out of its window of normal function becomes not an occasional counterbalancing mechanism but a nearly permanent condition—an on/off switch stuck almost always on "off." The effects on sexuality and many other aspects of the male metabolism are almost entirely negative.

Like so many things that work well when we're young, the control mechanism aspect of estrogen can get out of hand as we grow older. Illness, drugs, dietary imbalances, lifestyle, and certain aspects of normal aging help accelerate this process and raise estrogen levels to unhealthy heights. One of the first things we notice is that levels of aromatase, the testosterone-to-estrogen convertor, increase. This is, in part, because systems for controlling aromatase falter. In addition, methods of eliminating estrogen once it has been created decline. As a result, the typical middle-aged man becomes overestrogenized.

In most middle-aged men, the ratio of testosterone to estrogen is significantly altered. In a young man, a ratio that might have been 50 to 1 is now 20 to 1, or even 7 or 8 to 1. Normal, age-related testosterone decline is partly responsible for these transformative ratios, but increases in estrogen are frequently even more significant. This changing ratio of testosterone to estrogen is the key to understanding the metabolic andropause. And the metabolic andropause is in many, if not most, men, the chief contributor to the male menopause.

It's appropriate at this point to mention just a few of the harmful effects caused by estrogen.

First, there is the well known fact that estrogen causes increases in clotting factors as well as narrowing of the coronary arteries in men. Recent research has confirmed that high estrogen levels are associated with increased risk of heart attacks in males—the exact opposite of its effect in females, in whom it certainly has cardioprotective effects, dilating the coronaries, decreasing clotting factors and revving up the body's natural clot-busting system.

Not only does too much estrogen have a neutering effect on men, but so does too little testosterone. This makes it very significant, indeed, that in many men, high estrogen levels cause an actual slowdown in testosterone production. The mechanism of action is that the female hormone occupies some of the hypothalamic receptors for testosterone in the brain. The hypothalamus interprets this as if it were testosterone filling those receptor sites. The hypothalamus is tricked into acting as if testosterone levels in the body are high, and so it fails to send out the hormones that would tell the pituitary gland to stimulate testosterone production in the gonads. This is a form of the secondary hypogonadism that we discussed in the last chapter, dependent now not upon a disease state or pharmaceutical side effects or mere aging but purely upon an inappropriately high level of estrogen.

You'll see in just a few pages that there are still other negative effects that high estrogen has upon testosterone, but right now let's consider how estrogen gets high.

Seven Reasons for Estrogen Elevation

The most common causes of midlife estrogen increases in males are:

❏ Age-related increases in aromatase activity
❏ Alteration in liver function
❏ Zinc deficiency
❏ Obesity
❏ Overuse of alcohol
❏ Drug-induced estrogen inbalance
❏ Ingestion of estrogen-enhancing food or environmental substances

Almost all of these problems are interrelated, and one frequently reinforces or is the outright cause of another. Nonetheless, it's probably useful to look at them separately first.

Aromatase activity. First, there is aging itself. As a man grows older, he produces larger quantities of aromatase, the testosterone convertor. Consequently, he tends to convert higher levels of estrogen. It may well be that being overweight is the main reason for this apparently age-related change. If so, aromatase increase is controllable. If not, we can still take steps to minimize it.

Liver function. Alterations in liver function involve the important P450 system—a primary processing system that eliminates chemicals, hormones, drugs, and metabolic waste products from the body. Among its many duties is the task of excreting excess estrogen from the body. We will find that a wide variety of factors (including alcohol intake) can impair this system and tend to do so with age. In many individuals, this results in a gradual buildup of estrogen. In fact, the P450 system may be the most important factor in metabolic andropause.

Zinc deficiency. Zinc status is critical. Since zinc inhibits levels of aromatase, the testosterone-to-estrogen convertor, declining zinc will adversely affect the male/female hormone ratio. Inadequate levels of zinc are extremely common in the American diet, particularly among the elderly. In addition, alcohol, drugs (see the next page), and disease can significantly lower zinc levels. Zinc is also necessary for normal pituitary function, without which the proper hormonal signals will not be sent to the testicles to stimulate the production of testosterone. There is an interesting circular relationship here. Not only is zinc important for testosterone, but testosterone has been found to be necessary to maintain levels of zinc in the tissues.

Clearly in men whose zinc status is inadequate, the vicious cycle that becomes established must be broken into at some point through zinc supplementation.

Obesity. Next—whatever your sex—plumpness will tend to estrogenize you. Since fat cells contain aromatase, an increase in fat cell population will cause an increased testosterone-to-estrogen conversion rate. Moreover, obesity has been clearly associated with lower testosterone levels at all ages. It's not surprising, therefore, that overweight men almost invariably show signs of an unfavorable testosterone/estrogen ratio.

Alcohol use. Heavy alcohol intake also causes a dramatic rise in estrogen. Women, for instance, can increase their circulating estrogen levels threefold after just one drink. The rise in men is less dramatic but very significant nonetheless. Alcohol is closely related to two aspects of the problem we just discussed: it inhibits the P450 system, and it decreases zinc levels. Therefore, males who think that "real men" can hold their liquor and plenty of it have got it exactly wrong. Hormonally speaking, real men don't drink.

Alcohol and the Male

Heavy drinking in men has long been recognized as causing high estrogen levels with such related symptoms as spider veins, reddish coloration of the palms, gynecomastia (enlarged breasts), and even testicular atrophy. Increased sexual dysfunction is also common. Shakespeare noted that alcohol "increases the desire but decreases the performance," and there is every reason to believe that alcohol-induced estrogen rises are a significant part of that effect.

Drugs. Finally, a variety of prescription drugs have unfortunate effects. Perhaps the most common class of problem drug are the diuretics. Millions of American men are taking these "water" pills to treat high blood pressure. Though the effects on blood pressure are certainly good in the short term, long-term use of diuretics actually lowers life expectancy. I suspect one of the ways it does this is by removing sizable quantities of zinc from the body. As we noted earlier, this increases aromatase, and the long-term estrogen increases that result may cause more cardiovascular damage in men than the diuretics prevent. It is necessary to take fairly high doses of zinc (50 to 100 mg daily) to reverse these effects.

Caught in the Storm

You may think all this talk about estrogen, aromatase, P450 systems, etc. sounds relatively undramatic, but for the unfortunate man who is victimized by metabolic andropause, this network of hormonal effects combines to create a catastrophic whirlwind. These effects not only feed upon each other, they help to destroy the potency of testosterone.

Let's go back and consider again what part of testosterone is most significant in working the hormone's magic. You'll recall that there's something called free testosterone. That's the crucial slice of the total hormone pie. Total testosterone does not in any sense accurately represent the hormone's activity. Most of the 800 to 1200 ng/dl of testosterone found in young men is bound to other substances in the blood and not readily usable. Free testosterone—the unbound remainder—typically constitutes 2 to 3 percent of the whole. That 2 to 3 percent is hormonal gold, able to penetrate the cells of the body and command performance: strength in the muscles, potency in the gonads, energy in the mind, activity in all the cells and tissues where testosterone plays a role.

There are a number of substances in the bloodstream that bind testosterone and limit the amount of free testosterone. By far the most significant is a protein called sex hormone–binding globulin (SHBG). SHBG also increases with age, in all probability largely because of changes in our hormones. We know, for instance, that estrogen increases the body's production of SHBG. And high levels of testosterone actually depress production of SHBG.

It's clear, then, that a man with a high testosterone level and a low estrogen level will have less SHBG and will therefore keep a higher percentage of his total testosterone in the potent free form. Conversely, a man whose testosterone is declining will not only have less to start with but will bind a higher percentage of it to SHBG. And a man who is also experiencing higher estrogen levels will produce still more SHBG. As a result, in some individuals the percent of unbound testosterone available may be far less than the standard 2 to 3 percent.

The fact is a typical middle-aged man who wants to maintain an ideal hormonal balance is being hit hard on many fronts simultaneously. If he wants to remain slim, he should keep his testosterone level up, but, in fact, his testosterone level is probably declining. This predisposes him to weight gain. Weight gain increases his estrogen level and estrogen stimulates SHBG, which binds more testosterone, crippling the effectiveness of the hormone, which may cause more weight gain, which increases estrogen, and so on.

Moreover, if he drinks alcohol he reinforces the pattern. One of the main effects of alcohol is to turn down the P450 system in the liver. As we've already noted, that system is necessary to properly eliminate estrogen from the body. Meanwhile, age and perhaps a zinc deficiency has increased aromatase in his body and, consequently, more and more of his testosterone is being turned into estrogen. Which stimulates SHBG, which binds testosterone, which again repeats the cycle.

What I am proposing is far more dynamic and revolutionary than the old, simplistic view (I certainly held it myself for quite some time) in which male menopause is simply the result of lessened production of testosterone. Most men show a more complicated pattern of physical change. A more complicated problem usually requires a more complicated solution, and that's certainly the case here. As you're about to discover, additional testosterone may not even help the metabolically andropausal man. If his testosterone level goes up but his estrogen level goes up even faster, creating a worsening testosterone/estrogen ratio, then he may feel worse. Fortunately, there is a way around this problem. Otherwise, it would be necessary to accept the conclusion of many endocrinologists—that testosterone is useful only in a limited number of men. That turns out not to be the case because we can naturally alter the hormonal pathways and tap into the potential of the male hormone while quieting the rambunctious female hormone.

The Type of Replacement Matters

At this point, we discover that the mode of testosterone administration is all important. As I mentioned in the first chapter, probably no other type of hormone is replaced in the human body by so many different methods. When a man is suffering not merely from declining levels of testosterone but from metabolic andropause, he and his physician must carefully consider what method is right for him. Should he take shots, use creams, put on a patch, or have a pellet implanted in his buttock?

Men whose andropausal problem revolves around an excess conversion of testosterone to estrogen will usually find that the last two methods are most appropriate. Studies in the treatment of impotence and other andropausal conditions that do not report high levels of success with testosterone almost invariably administer the hormone through injection. What typically happens when an andropausal man receives an injection of testosterone is that his testosterone levels rise sharply, and he feels a significant improvement at first. In a relatively short time, however, a sizable proportion of the hormone is converted to estrogen by aromatase. The consequent effects upon both the man's energy level and his sex life are usually quite negative.

The treatment has caused an unfavorable shift in the estrogen/testosterone ratio. Let us suppose that a typical fifty-five-year-old male started with a testosterone level of 460 ng/dl and an estrogen level of 20 ng/dl. A few days after his injection, tests will show that his testosterone—which might have gone as high as 1200 ng/dl in the twenty-four hours after he first received the replacement dose—has stabilized at 840 ng/dl. It's a good level and ought to have him feeling fine. Unfortunately, so much of that initial high surge of testosterone got converted to estrogen that—*if you test for estrogen, and most doctors don't*—you may find that his estrogen has gone up to 60 ng/dl.

In a case like that, the initial estrogen/testosterone ratio was 1 to 23. The new ratio is 1 to 14. And the ratio of estrogen to free testosterone may be even worse. In fact, the poor man may have even less free testosterone now than he had before he started, even though his total testosterone has nearly doubled. Remember total testosterone is not very important; free testosterone is crucial. And increases in estrogen are likely to play havoc with free testosterone by increasing the amount of sex hormone–binding globulin, which binds it up.

It seems that the reason why testosterone injections and, to a lesser extent, testosterone creams cause such estrogen increases is that they temporarily—when first administered—drive testosterone up into an unusually high, nonphysiologic range. For reasons that we don't entirely know, this causes a significant conversion to estrogen. Fortunately, the other two methods—the testosterone patch and pellet implantation—release testosterone into the body in slow, steady doses and don't normally cause large increases in estrogen.

Finding the Balance

Let's watch this process in a real person.

David B. had reached the age of fifty-eight, after years of success in the highly competitive field of aerospace engineering. David had loved the work, had made many innovations, had had quite a career over the years. Now he felt he was coming unstuck. He woke up every morning unrested, his memory was playing tricks, his mental concentration came and went in fits and starts. At home he was irritable, depressed, and sexually out to lunch. David's self-confidence was shattered.

When I checked his hormone levels, I found a marginal testosterone level of 365 ng/dl and a very high estrogen of 52 ng/dl. I tried David at first on testosterone patches, but his testosterone only went up to 520 ng/dl and his estrogen rose a little more to 58 ng/dl. We had to get his estrogen down. I started giving David zinc and soy protein. He felt a little better, but he drank four or five beers a day. I asked him to cut it to two.

That did the trick. David is functioning quite well now with a testosterone level in the 500s and an estrogen level that generally stays around 30 ng/dl. His mental concentration has come back, the crushing fatigue that used to follow him through the day is gone. At home, his sexual interest has returned.

I hope we can get David to feel even better. If he would improve his diet and start to get a little exercise, I know it would make a difference. Nonetheless, David is fully alive again. He's a very typical case of the most basic treatment for metabolic andropause.

CHAPTER 6:
The Key to Male Sexuality

Few subjects fascinate the human mind more than sex. Blazing through our lives at puberty, eventually settling down a little as we settle down, it still holds our interest as the years pile on. Most of us would like to keep the glow of desire and desirability as long as we live.

That can make it difficult for middle-aged men because in midlife, a surprisingly high number of them see their sexual capacity diminishing—at first, perhaps, subtly—then, all too often, drastically. They don't know what to do about it, and many, if not most men are far too appalled to discuss it with anyone, including their doctor.

That's an awful dilemma, not only because sexual function can usually be brought back to normal, but because sexual malfunctioning, even in its earliest stages, is a tip-off that other health changes are emerging. Those may be fraught with significant or lethal consequence. Sexual change can forecast heart disease and diabetes, conditions common in the male menopause. The extent to which you're at risk naturally depends upon your individual genetics, not to mention diet, exercise, lifestyle—the whole personalized ball of wax. Sexual change, nonetheless, is a message from your body, not infrequently a message about cardiovascular changes. Things *down there* point a finger toward the future.

I'm going to concentrate in this chapter on sexual decline in males, especially as manifested by erectile malfunction. Outright sexual failure—impotence—is very rare in young males. By midlife it becomes much more frequent; also, other aspects of sexuality, such as length of time required to attain an erection, the force of ejaculation, the amount of ejaculate, the degree of pleasure, the rigidity of the erection, change markedly, even in men who, strictly speaking, don't have potency problems. Naturally, these changes are interconnected and related to the likelihood of eventual erectile dysfunction.

I'm going to take a largely hormonal approach to male sexuality and potency here. For a discussion of certain other approaches, see Appendix 1. They can be important, too.

That being said, I can't stress too strongly the overwhelming significance of testosterone for creating and maintaining the virile functioning of the male sexual organs. Many endocrinologists and urologists these days have been influenced by prevalent misconceptions about testosterone created by drastically flawed studies. In the medical literature, it has been widely published that only 5 percent of sexual dysfunction can be treated hormonally. In fact, the majority of sexual dysfunction has a vital hormonal component and, if caught early, can be corrected with hormones. The earlier the intervention occurs, the less likely the damage is to be permanent.

The major points this chapter will address are as follows:

❑ The relationship of testosterone to the structural and functional integrity of the male organ.

❑ The precise physical elements that make an erection possible.

❑ The evidence of animal studies for the effectiveness of the hormonal approach.

❑ The reason that potency experts have underestimated the effectiveness of a hormonal approach.

❑ The role of estrogen.

❑ The lessons that my patients taught me.

❑ The significance of nitric oxide and the relationship of cardiovascular function to sex function.

So much for our summary. Now, let's look at the basic reasons that testosterone rules in the kingdom of the male genitals.

Testosterone Is in Charge Down Here

If testosterone doesn't have a major role to play in making every-thing down there work properly, then the design of the human body must be grossly inefficient, because everything in the genital/pelvic region that could affect the functioning of the penis is packed with testosterone receptors. I'm sure you recall the description in Chapter 4 of how, in the second month after con-ception, the male sexual organs begin to form due to the effects of the testosterone that was secreted from the genital ridge. In fact, all the different structural components of the genital area—nerves, arteries, veins, muscles—are guided in their formation by testosterone and maintained in good, working order, throughout life, by that very same hormone. At puberty, the very start of our potential and desire for an active sex life, surges of testosterone alter us permanently, as we've all observed. Sexual desire appears

Table 3: *Effects of Aging on Male Sexual Function*

Mental arousal

Cortical response to sensory stimuli	Decreased

Physical arousal

Penile sensitivity	Decreased
Neural response to stimuli	Slower
Sense of impending orgasm	Decreased

Orgasm

Ejaculatory force	Decreased
Semen volume and viscosity	Decreased
Scrotal and testicular elevation	Decreased
Prostate contractions	Decreased
Urethral contractions	Decreased

Refractory period

Time before next arousal	Longer
Postejaculatory detumescence	Quicker

along with growth of the sexual organs and a grand display of the secondary sexual attributes that contribute so vividly to differentiating the sexes and exciting their mutual admiration.

All this happens, of course, because testosterone plugs into the receptors that are avidly awaiting its arrival and causes the whole shebang to light up. The male hormone goes on doing that right through a healthy male's life.

The truth is that the muscles, the nerves, and the arteries and veins (the vascular system) in the pelvic/genital region of a man's body need testosterone stimulation to function, will not function for long without it, and, in the majority of cases, can—after testosterone deprivation—be restored to function if testosterone is restored. Testosterone is *numero uno* just where it counts the most. This is quite a picture of hormone essentiality, and it's very different from what you'll hear if you go to a typical potency specialist. Let me also say in passing—more will be said a little further on—that other sex hormones have a role to play in the genital area. The enzyme for converting testosterone to dihydrotestosterone and the aromatase enzyme that the body uses to convert testosterone to estrogen are both found there in fairly substantial quantities. They, too, have critical roles to play.

Now, let's pause and take a look at the mechanics of genital sexuality in the male.

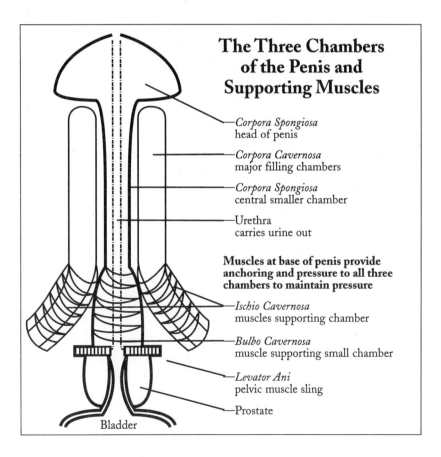

The Three Chambers of the Penis and Supporting Muscles

Corpora Spongiosa
head of penis

Corpora Cavernosa
major filling chambers

Corpora Spongiosa
central smaller chamber

Urethra
carries urine out

Muscles at base of penis provide anchoring and pressure to all three chambers to maintain pressure

Ischio Cavernosa
muscles supporting chamber

Bulbo Cavernosa
muscle supporting small chamber

Levator Ani
pelvic muscle sling

Prostate

Bladder

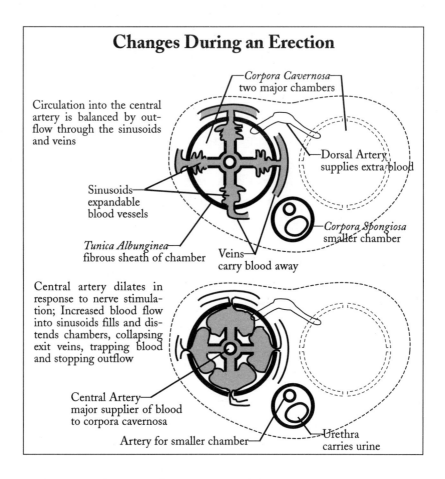

Changes During an Erection

Circulation into the central artery is balanced by out-flow through the sinusoids and veins

—Corpora Cavernosa— two major chambers

—Dorsal Artery supplies extra blood

Sinusoids— expandable blood vessels

—Corpora Spongiosa smaller chamber

Tunica Albunginea— fibrous sheath of chamber

Veins— carry blood away

Central artery dilates in response to nerve stimulation; Increased blood flow into sinusoids fills and distends chambers, collapsing exit veins, trapping blood and stopping outflow

Central Artery— major supplier of blood to corpora cavernosa

Artery for smaller chamber—

—Urethra carries urine

What Makes Doing It Doable

As a sexual tool, the penis is remarkably complex and elegantly effective. If it's to enlarge and stiffen sufficiently to permit penetration, three different systems must play a part. The nervous system must receive and send signals, the vascular system must supply sufficient blood to fill the penile chambers, and the muscular system in those lower regions of the body must exert pressures allowing the erection to be created and maintained. Without all of these systems working together, a normal, functioning erection is not in the cards.

Erections begin as a result of the stimulation of the nervous system. This can occur in many different ways, but all of the communications are filtered through the brain. Even the direct sensory stimulation of the genital organs will send messages along the pudendal nerve and up the spine to the central nervous system message centers. Everything else gets there, too. Sexual feelings, verbal or visual communications with the loved one, touching and kissing, or, if a man is by himself, erotic fantasy, sexual imagery, anticipation, memory, or any other excitation of desire will each in its turn stimulate various regions of the brain. All these regions combine their messages in the hypothalamus, from whence the good news is sent southwards in a cascade of neurotransmitter signals. Certain parts of the message go directly down the spinal cord to the penis. But the autonomic nervous system, that which controls unconscious functions of the body such as breathing and digesting, also receives the message and transmits it through chemical signals that the entire body responds to. So an extraordinary variety of incoming stimuli—everything from the words, "I love you," to the gentle touch of a loving hand—combine to send a variety of neuronal signals towards the groin, all with an essentially similar message: "Attention, please!"

The penis is, of course, primed to respond to the signals the body is so eager to send it. A man's sexual organ is a pretty unusual piece of equipment, basically an inflatable, multichambered filling tank with a slender tube running down its center. No other part of either the male or the female body carries out at short notice such an extraordinary transformation as the penis.

Triggered by stimuli from the central nervous system and/or the peripheral nervous system, the muscular walls of the arteries dilate allowing more blood to flow into the genital region. As that blood arrives, the smooth muscles in the penis relax, so that the penile chambers can grow to their full capacity. The penis has three of these spongelike cavities. The most important are the two *corpora cavernosa*, twin cylinders that run lengthwise up and down the penis on each side of the urethra. The third chamber, the *corpus spongiosum*, is a continuous group of spongy blood vessels that run down the length of the organ, expanding at the top to form the head, or glans, of the penis.

Once the blood vessels dilate, the blood flows into the chambers through the central and dorsal arteries. There, the smaller arterioles, which form the mesh or plexus of interconnecting vessels, rapidly dilate to form sinusoids, or swollen poolings of blood. The relatively firm though stretchable tissue that forms the outer layer of the *corpora cavernosa*—surrounding each chamber like a glove—readily expands to contain these poolings of arterial blood; so readily that an erect penis contains eight times as much blood as a flaccid one. Engorged with blood, the penis is rigid, and the veins that would normally carry the blood away are compressed between the spongelike tissue of the cavernosa and the fibrous sheath that forms their outer wall, so that now only small amounts of blood escape.

While all of this is going on, the whole package is firmly held together by the muscles of the pelvic sling—the *levator ani*. Some of these muscles are specifically assigned to the task of anchoring the penis and supporting its three filling chambers. Without exercise and lifelong hormonal support, these muscles grow weak. In all honesty, the neglect of this muscular component of erectile function is one of the most astonishing failures of current clinical practice in the field of impotence. Look at the following sidebar for an extended discussion of these muscles.

The whole process is quite efficient, and, in a young male, the time that it takes to produce an erection can be measured in seconds. Once created, an erect penis ought to be able to maintain its state until either ejaculation or an interruption in sexual excitement occurs. Though complex, it sounds like a very workable system. Why does it decline? Why does the impotency rate in young men stand at around 1 percent and the impotency rate in seventy-year-olds exceed 30 percent? I believe the answer is largely hormonal.

What happens in the nerves, the vascular system, and the muscles connected to the penis when a man's testosterone supply drys up? Well, just consider.

The *Levator Ani* Muscles

This unattractively named set of muscles (the Latin refers to "lifting the anus") are the background music to most of the sexual delights you've experienced. They form a large, muscular hammock or sling across the bottom of the pelvis—from stem to stern.

The *levator ani* muscles are even more dependent on testosterone than most other skeletal muscle groups. The area is packed with testosterone receptors, and, consequently, any shortage of the male hormone will cause a swift decline in muscle tone and contractile properties down there. This results in a general atrophy and thinning of the muscle fibers.

Just what are these muscles designed to do?

Envision the broad fibers of the *levator ani* muscle forming a basket-like or hammock-like sling from the pubic bone in the front to the sacrum and coccyx, or tailbone, in the rear. In men and women, there are further specialized muscle bundles that spin off from the basket to form circular, napkin ring-like muscle groups called sphincters. These maintain constant tone to prevent loss of urine or feces/gas, etc., in between occasions of normal voiding or defecating. What a job! Imagine holding back the floodgates of embarrassing emissions during every cough, laugh, or misstep we make. Try jumping up and down—but don't do it without a healthy *levator ani* sling! Just ask any woman with a leaky bladder. Loss of androgen effect results in loss of full muscle tone—which causes spurts, dribbles, leaks, stains, and gas.

(Continued on next page)

(Continued from previous page)

Let's stick with the men. In their case, starting from the bones we sit on, called the ischial tuberosities, two critical muscles extend their support and anchor the penis. The first of these muscles is called the *ischio cavernosa*. Its fiberous muscular layers surround the main filling chambers of the penis, the *corpora cavernosa*, at their base. We've described how, when triggered by nerve stimuli, the smooth muscles of the arteries contract opening the flow into the chambers through the central and dorsal arteries.

The *ischio cavernosa* muscles surrounding the base of the chambers both anchor the chambers and provide additional tension to the outer fibrous membrane, which helps to maintain the necessary compression of the vessels during the various pressures of intercourse.

After climax, the nerve tone rapidly decreases resulting in arterial constriction and rapid decompression of the chambers, allowing for veins to redilate and carry away the exhausted but happy red blood cells so they can be recharged in the lungs.

There is also a second muscle affecting the function of the penis. Surrounding the urethra where it enters the penis, this is called the *bulbo cavernosa* muscle. This muscle has its own nerve and blood supply and contributes an additional and vital force to erectal function. As we've seen, the blood vessels surrounding the urethra also form a mesh or network that expands at the end to form the head of the penis and is called the *corpus spongiosum*. This third chamber fills more by constriction of the muscle fibers surrounding it than by compression of the veins. The griplike pressure of the *bulbo cavernosa* muscle has a chokehold on this blood supply—don't let go or deflating pressure can lead to a hang-your-head experience.

The *bulbo cavernosa* muscle can actually be flexed when a man has an erection, causing the head of the penis to jerk upwards. As men get older, the erect penis tends to hang at a lower angle, no longer jutting out stiffly upright. This change results from weakening of the *bulbo cavernosa*. This muscle also controls the propelling of semen out of the storage chambers and through the urethra with strong pulsating contractions. Therefore, less forceful and pleasurable ejaculations can generally be traced back to a weakening of the *bulbo cavernosa*.

What maintains the conditioning of this vital muscle? Testosterone! Without hormonal input, the muscle gradually withers and sustained fullness of the erection becomes impossible. Even more catastrophically, decrease the tension of the *ischio cavernosis* muscle that surrounds and supports the corpus cavernosa and blood will not be maintained in the chambers, with results as deflating to the ego as a flat tire in the Indianapolis 500.

Without Testosterone the System Atrophies

We know from animal studies that without testosterone the muscle, nerve, and vascular systems that a man's sexual organs depend on grow weak. In male rats, both the muscles and the nerves in the groin have high levels of androgen receptors—just as men have. When the rats are castrated, the muscle fibers in their levator ani rapidly weaken. Moreover, the nerve endings in the pelvic region alter and cease to transmit messages effectively. The poor rat has been hormonally torched; he soon loses the capacity to produce an erection. If researchers had any doubts that these carefully observed changes in structure and function were due to the loss of testosterone, the doubts were put to rest by further experiment. When the castrated rats were given testosterone even months after castration, they gradually began to regenerate both the muscles and nerves that had atrophied so swiftly after the loss of their testicles. In fact, nerve and muscle function were brought back to almost 100 percent, and sexual desire and capability returned.[1]

Clearly, in rodents, all those testosterone receptors weren't put in the pelvic region for naught.

Why Hasn't Testosterone Worked for Urologists?

Testosterone has worked for my patients, as you'll momentarily see. Why hasn't it worked for urologists or for the researchers whose studies have discouraged most physicians treating impotence from turning to the male hormone?

There are, of course, a variety of reasons. Even I, with my enthusiasm for hormonal solutions and my very satisfactory clinical track record, have to admit two things: rats are not people, and not every man gets erectile function back after hormone administration.

We are, of course, a great deal more complex than rodents, even though the structure of the genital organs and testosterone's effects on them are very similar in all mammals. People, however, live much longer, suffer more complicated patterns of cardiovascular decline, and do things a rat would never dream of doing. People take drugs (see Appendix 3), especially antihypertensives and anticonvulsants that directly damage erectile function. They smoke—one of the surest fire methods of injuring the blood vessels in the penis. They drink—an established downer. They become obese—bad for the muscles, bad for the estrogen level, bad for potency. They suffer from diabetes and heart disease, although, as you'll see in the next chapter, proper treatment for these pervasive ills can include a vigorous hormonal approach. Nevertheless, it is a fact that blood vessel weakness can lead to an incapacity to fill those pooling chambers in the penis.

All of this is my way of admitting that, though I have seen a high percentage of sexual recoveries after a properly administered program of testosterone, there's no such thing as a foolproof therapy. Some patients are unfortunately too far gone sexually for a benign hormonal approach to work. But bear in mind, these folks are in the minority.

Which still leaves us with the question of why so many medical professionals are unaware of the successes they could be achieving with testosterone.

Part of the answer seems to be our old friend estrogen. The genital receptors that function so well when testosterone lights their fire can also be occupied by estrogen molecules. As you've already seen, when testosterone is administered by injection very high levels are often reached within the first few days, and this frequently results in a rapid conversion of a portion of that testosterone to estrogen. Some estrogen is, of course, necessary even in males. That's why we have an enzyme to create it. In fact, males who have a genetic defect depriving them of aromatase are generally found to be without sexual desire although their sexual organs are apparently functional. The question is always one of balance. There is a window within which estrogen levels are, more or less, ideal. Once out of that window, problems occur. Certainly, if the estrogen level rises too high, then receptor sites that were ready and eager to receive the male hormone are blocked by the female. This is not an ideal prescription for male virility. Is it coincidental that a study done in 1988 at UCLA found that the most significant hormonal association with impotence was high estrogen?[2]

Let's look at two cases that may clarify this situation somewhat.

Two Cases That Brought Me to the Crossroads

Warren M. was a patient I had followed over the years, although he was being managed by the urologist who had treated him for testicular cancer. After a recurrence of cancer in his second testicle (necessitating its removal), Warren—now in his early forties—was left without a source of testosterone and was put on testosterone by his urologist. Warren got 400 mg in the butt every month, a standard dose at that time and still popular today. As I would occasionally do the injection, I was naturally curious about its efficacy.

To my surprise, Warren reported that the shot only worked well for a week then wore off. In the third week, he found himself "getting horny again" for a few days, and then the effects faded completely in the week before his next injection. A rollercoaster in reverse order. I was puzzled by this pattern but felt that probably there had been damage to his reflexes from radiation therapy done after his first cancer.

Still, why was the effect the lowest when the shot was peaking in his blood stream and higher toward the end? Reflecting that it is not given to doctors to understand everything about their patients (or even their own therapies), I advised Warren to hang in there, that time was the great healer. He stuck in my mind as a curiosity—that is, until Harold came along.

Harold T. was sixty, a successful businessman who had been a pretty good athlete most of his life. At the country club tennis courts nearby where Harold lived, he had been known for his cannonball serve and hard play at the net. But no more. The strength, stamina, and quickness were no longer there. Harold was being beaten by people he had handled easily in the past.

Sex had always been an important thing for Harold, too. He thought of himself as a pretty good lover. No more of that either. For some years now, he had been watching his sex function and desire decline together. By the time he reached sixty, the hard fact was he was basically impotent—Harold hadn't had a successful, sustainable erection in more than a year.

He came to see me looking pretty grim. He wanted his energy and his sexual prowess back again. I told him we'd check his hormone levels. His testosterone was 396 ng/dl, within the official definition of normal but not by much. I suspected that, with an athletic fellow like Harold, this represented a highly significant decline. His estrogen was 44 ng/dl, a little high. I started giving Harold testosterone shots—200 mg every two weeks.

At his next visit, he told me his energy was coming back, and he was starting to experience some sexual twinges that he interpreted very positively. Approximately a month after we started treatment, Harold was potent for the first time. I don't have to tell you how he looked when he came in and told me that. A few weeks later, however, there was the first inkling of dissatisfaction. He seemed sexually quiescent, off his stride. Harold wanted to know if I could increase the dose. I did.

There was a slight improvement, followed by a further relapse. Harold said how about more, and I said let's check your hormone levels again. His testosterone was up to 730 ng/dl, but his estrogen had increased to 90 ng/dl. This was a crossroads for me—it was the first time that I fully realized what the increases in estrogen were doing. I had my first inkling of why some men didn't do well with injections.

Eventually I gave Harold the full anti-estrogen program with 50 mg of zinc twice daily, hefty quantities of soy protein in his diet, and avoidance of alcohol. After some experimentation, I put him on time-release pellets of testosterone. This gives lower amounts of testosterone at steady levels and tends not to provoke large upsurges of estrogen. The next time I measured Harold's blood levels, his testosterone was 656 ng/dl, and his estrogen was 35 ng/dl. The balance was now far better. To strengthen Harold's pelvic area, I set him to work doing Kegel exercises.

And Harold's smiles soon returned. Within two months his sexual encounters were successful more often than not and improvement continued from there. A year after I first saw him, Harold reported that sex was better now than it had been in a decade. His erectile difficulties were a thing of the past. And, as if that wasn't enough, his strength, energy, and athletic ability had also staged a resurgence.

What was happening to Harold? It was quite clear to me that his genital organs and the whole pelvic region that supports them were just waiting to receive the hormonal signal to light up. The same thing was true of the muscles that gave him his athleticism.

If you've looked at the boxes on pages 67 and 68, you've seen how important I believe muscles to be when it comes to supporting a man's capacity to perform sexually. One of the many flaws in the impotence studies that failed to attach due significance to testosterone replacement was that they gave testosterone for a relatively short time and simply expected it to magically induce potency—as if it were an anti-impotency drug. But, of course, it's not a drug at all, it's a body-building hormone. And body building is an active process, not simply a passive reception of treatment. A young man won't become muscular just by sitting on his high hormone levels. He has to go out and exercise! Body builders don't form their exceptional musculature simply by taking steroids (which, alas, many of them do); they lift weights and challenge their muscles on exercise machines.

So, if you've have had erectile difficulties, don't simply find a physician to prescribe testosterone. Read Appendix 2 carefully, and do some Kegel exercises.

Eventually . . .

Harold got fairly quick results. I've known other patients who didn't see any significant sexual improvement for at least six months to a year. The degenerative process that causes the decline of muscles, blood vessels, and nerves occurs over many, many years. Like so many of the other physical ills precipitated by hormone decline as we age, it is practically a lifetime project. Rebuilding erectile function, therefore, can easily be a major program involving a major investment of time and effort.

Some fortunate males who read this passage today will say, "I'm not sure I know what you're talking about, Dr. Shippen. I'm fifty-five, and I don't feel much of this 'gradual decline.' I'm potent and happy and strong!" My answer is, "I believe you, but just wait."

The male menopause comes to all of us. But unlike the female menopause, it certainly doesn't come on schedule. The timetable for this change of life hasn't been printed. Some men are deep in the thick of it by the time they're fifty, and others—a happy few—might almost wonder what you're talking about if you mention it to them when they're seventy-five.

One patient of mine, Winwood F., reminds me of just how much variability male sexuality can have. Winwood was my patient for a long time before we ever discussed sexuality. Eventually—when he was eighty-three—I heard the whole story. Winwood and his wife had had a normal sex life until their mid-fifties. Then the effects of cancer surgery and postsurgical radiation had made intercourse too painful for her. For the next fifteen years, Winwood lived a celibate life. He told me it hadn't been too difficult for him; he got used to it and had occasional nocturnal emissions. His wife died when he was seventy-one, and two years later he acquired a girlfriend and rediscovered his sex life. For the next ten years, he and his she vigorously frolicked in the haystacks. Then, at the age of eighty-three, Winwood came to me with two complaints. For the past six months to a year, he had been feeling increasingly fatigued and his sex life had gone rapidly downhill. I put him on testosterone (I gave him shots, and fortunately Winwood didn't produce much estrogen), and everything straightened out. So much so that when I asked him about his sex life, he smiled slyly and said, "Oh, that—I got an erection you could have hung a paint bucket on." That was four years ago, and, at eighty-seven, Winwood F. and his girlfriend are still trucking—and he's still taking his hormones.

What we're seeing here, of course, is the coming of the male menopause. Only, in Winwood's case, it didn't arrive until his eighties.

What Should a Man Think? What Should He Do?

In the old days, if a man found he wasn't feeling as much desire as he used to and the sexual apparatus wasn't functioning with the predictability or the forcefulness that he customarily expected, he set it down to his years: "Oh, well I must be getting older." By and large, that's true, but now we know that the type of getting older that occurs is, for the most part, hormonal.

A discussion of other approaches to treating sexual and erectile decline is found in Appendix 1. If you're seeing a doctor, you should also keep in mind some of the testosterone-lowering conditions in the following table that are not necessarily age related.

Table 4: *Factors that Lower Testosterone and Raise Impotence*

COPD/hypoxia

asthma

corticosteroid use

presence of cancer

cancer chemotherapy

obesity

malnutrition

critical illness

If you do desire to improve your sexual function through testosterone replacement, keep the following points in mind.

1) Both testosterone and estrogen levels should be measured. If estrogen begins or becomes too high, it may be necessary to follow some of the suggestions outlined in Chapter 5.

2) Patches or pellets are usually superior therapies; they provide a slower, steadier supply of testosterone, and they are much less prone to incite estrogen increases.

3) If you're on prescription (especially the ones in Appendix 3), you'll need to work with your physician to determine whether they are affecting your sex function; if they are, it may be possible to change the drugs or alter the dosage.

4) It is probably advisable to practice Kegel exercises to improve muscle tone in the pelvic area. See Appendix 2. In one British study, the exercises *alone* were just as effective as surgery (yuck!) in correcting impotence.[3]

5) Be patient and persistent. Hormonal treatment is not a lightning bolt. It took you a long time to lose the sexual function with which you began. It may take you as long as a year to get it back.

From the Penis to the Heart

The last thing I want to discuss in this chapter is the one aspect of erectile function that we may have given short shrift to so far. Obviously no erection occurs without a massive flow of blood into the penis. If any doctors reading this chapter feel tempted to criticize my optimistic estimation of the effects of testosterone, they will probably do so on the grounds that I have not adequately accounted for the negative effects of cardiovascular deterioration on penile function.

There's little doubt that they have a case. If age-related or smoking-related or diabetes-related atherosclerosis has progressed so far that normal blood flow to the penis is compromised, then potency may be difficult to restore. But frankly, my experience has been that, the majority of time, restoration can occur. The principle reason, I believe, is that testosterone is not only an essential part of the male sexual system but is, as well, a significant element in the recovery of cardiovascular function.

In fact, a sizable number of recent medical studies show testosterone to be one of the major stimulators of nitric oxide.[4] This has broad significance for testosterone's role in promoting both erectile function and cardiovascular health. Nitric oxide is a neurotransmitter that stimulates the nerves, causing erection and also vasodilation, i.e., relaxation and improved blood flow in the major cardiovascular blood vessels such as the aorta.[5]

Could it be that there is a powerful relationship between a man's sexual function and his heart health? We have more and more reason to think so. Potency experts have long used a comparison between blood pressure in the penis and in the arm, the so-called penial/brachial ratio, as an index of erectile force and function. Ideally, the ratio should be one-to-one. If the blood pressure in the arm is found to be significantly higher than the pressure in the penis, then the outlook for erectile health isn't bright. Recently, however, researchers have discovered that a low penial/brachial ratio also correlates with a high risk for heart attacks and strokes.[6] What could that mean? I think the next chapter will give you the answer.

CHAPTER 7:

Testosterone and Your Heart

Stanford R. is seventy-four years old now, but he has had heart problems since the early 1970s. It didn't make life easy for him. He's an athletic man who likes to hunt, fish on the river, and walk in the woods. By the time Stanford, together with his chest pains, got into the 1980s, it was time for a quintuple bypass. The chest pains started up again a few years later. He was on lots of meds, his energy was down, his sex drive quiescent. But in the 1990s, Stan was put on a new approach. His chest pains went away, his energy returned, and, when he isn't out walking over the hills and fields and hunting in the woods, Stanford makes love. Sometimes twice a day.

The difference? The difference was testosterone, nothing more, nothing less.

If you're a man with heart problems, you must bring this chapter to the attention of your physician.

We don't normally regard the heart as a sex organ—except metaphorically—but you can be sure of one thing: testosterone, that preeminent male "sex hormone," is one of the most essential guardians of a healthy male heart. It plugs into the heart, hormone to receptor, as firmly as a lightbulb screws into a socket.

Why is this the case? We could hazard many quesses. For instance, testosterone is a muscle-building hormone, and the heart is the hardest working muscle in the human body. Muscle and hormone should be logically compelled to forge a connection. They do. In fact, there are more cellular sites for receiving testosterone in the human heart than in any other muscle of the human anatomy! If the number of receptors indicates the relative importance of a hormone, then the heart is certainly the major muscular target for testosterone.

Carrying this concept further, if testosterone is integral to normal function, then testosterone deficiency must result in some decrement in function, some pathologic change. Well, not only is testosterone the body's strongest factor for maintaining muscle protein, but, as a stimulator of arterial dilation, testosterone controls and increases production of nitric oxide, a natural form of nitroglycerin, the tablets heart patients take to open up the coronary arteries when angina pains arise. It's not surprising that the pumping power of the heart decreases when testosterone declines and that angina pains begin when nitric oxide production also declines. As we shall soon see these effects can be reversed when testosterone is restored.

An even more intriguing indication of the essential role of testosterone to the heart is the long list of risk factors for heart disease profoundly affected by the hormone. Scouring the medical literature provided me with a truckload of references to the relationship between testosterone and the heart. Most of them are not mentioned in lectures or at meetings of the American Heart Association, nor has anyone drawn them together into a unified concept. How often does one hear of a physician ordering a testosterone level when a patient comes in with cardiac complaints? Well, after they finish this chapter, most patients will demand it.

The fundamental fact is this: a clear and ever-increasing majority of medical studies report an association between high testosterone and low cardiovascular disease in men. This is not a coincidental association, since when testosterone is diminished well-accepted risk factors increase, and when testosterone is administered in appropriate doses *most of the major risk factors for heart disease diminish*. Moreover, in the majority of patients, symptoms and objective EKG measurements improve. These studies are confirming the results I have been getting with patients for years. Men prosper healthwise and live longer when their testosterone levels are normal. Heart problems, in particular, are more easily controlled.

Why hasn't testosterone been given a prominent role in the treatment of heart disease? The neglect is utterly puzzling, considering the depth of the research supporting its significance.

In the next ten or fifteen pages, I hope to convince you of one simple fact: if you're a man, there is an intimate connection between maintaining a relatively youthful testosterone level and remaining free of heart disease. It would be simplistic to say you can't have one without the other, but such an extravagant statement of the connection between this hormone and heart health would be closer to the truth than medicine has been willing to admit.

Turning the Popular Wisdom on Its Head

Of course, the statements I've just made reverse the mythology about testosterone that used to surface now and then in the popular press. Men, of course, do have far more heart attacks at an earlier age than women do—and, somewhere along the line, journalists and even doctors started saying that was because of the male hormone. However, there wasn't a shred of evidence to support that assumption.

The only way to defeat a myth is to supplant it with a strong body of fact. So, consider the following cardiovascular risk factors which *increase* as testosterone *decreases*:

❑ Cholesterol and triglyceride levels go up, leading to increased arterial plaque[1]
❑ Coronary artery and major artery dilation diminish—hence vasoconstriction and greater risk of cardiac events[2]
❑ Rising blood pressure[3]
❑ Increased insulin output, which leads to obesity, elevated blood pressure, adult diabetes, and increased cortisone output[4]
❑ Increased central abdominal fat; increased waist/hip ratio[5]
❑ Increased estrogen levels in men—associated with higher stroke and heart attack rates[6]
❑ Increased lipoprotein A[7]
❑ Increased fibrinogen—the basis of most blood clots (combined with a simultaneous drop in plasminogen, our natural clot buster)[8]
❑ Decreased human growth hormone (HGH) output, leading to a decline in energy, strength, stamina, and heart muscle mass and output[9]
❑ Decreased energy and strength, causing decreased physical activity thereby leading to obesity—the vicious cycle of the male menopause[10]

No other single factor in the male body that we know of correlates with more risk factors for heart disease than testosterone. It is like a central point around which the outstanding indicators of health or cardiovascular catastrophe whirl endlessly. Although the fashion in risk factors alters subtly and continuously, with cholesterol up in one decade and then down in the next while insulin or homocysteine or central body obesity, by contrast, rise, one stubborn fact remains. Only a very small minority of men get heart disease without first showing some of the laboratory indicators, the so-called "risk factors" shown here.

A nonsmoking man at his ideal weight with low cholesterol, normal triglyceride, normal blood pressure, as well as ideal homocysteine, fibrinogen, and insulin levels does not generally die of premature heart disease.

Since, by and large, all these risk factors show themselves on their best behavior when testosterone is high, we can be forgiven for assuming that there is something about testosterone that makes it protective. Perhaps, indeed, there is something about it which is purposefully built to save the lucky male who retains it at high levels from the perils of heart disease.

This chapter is designed to do nothing more than convince you that testosterone is the heart-protective hormone of the male body and that it can be used to protect you from the major killer of men and perhaps to rescue you from its clutches, if you already suffer cardiovascular impairment.

Testosterone works protectively in men, just as estrogen does for women; estrogen dominance for women, testosterone dominance for men. I think this is a clear case of Nature knowing what she's doing. But Nature is also cruel. She forges a clear link between the sexual vitality of her creatures and their ability to go on surviving. Once you reach the age at which sex hormones naturally begin a steep decline, you are also old enough for Nature to reach some rather grim conclusions about your importance. Basically, Nature makes the rather down and dirty assumption that your continued existence will not have significant survival benefits for the human race. You have probably had a chance to bear or sire children. You have been able to attend to the most crucial years of their upbringing. Your task is done. It would now be quite superfluous to use sex hormones to protect you any longer. Sex hormone levels, therefore, can be allowed to decline, because, if a heart attack kills a sixty-year-old, that—in Nature's scheme of things—is no great tragedy.

We humans adopt a different point of view—and we are not inclined to accept without a struggle Nature's plan of hormonal deprivation and ultimate fatal decline.

One of my patients, Ronald K., an eighty-year-old former truck driver, is a good example. Since the early 1980s, Ronald had heart problems with high blood pressure, severe chest pain, and occasional transient ischemic attacks (TIAs, which are mini-strokes). The medicines he took for his conditions made him weaker and weaker until, as he put it, "I didn't have enough ambition to get out of bed in the morning."

Ronald had pain when he went up the stairs and pain when he walked down the street. He gave up sex as too dangerous, even if he had been able to work up the interest anymore. His life was declining into a slow motion perambulation from the medicine chest to the refrigerator to the television set, and back home to bed at night.

In 1994 I started Ronald on testosterone, and, in less than four months, he was physically a different person. His chest pain went away, and he started taking walks. Ronald now walks a mile a day. Gradually, as his energy returned and his symptoms relented, Ronald's fear began to go away, too, and about six months after I put him on testosterone, he started making love again.

In the three and a half years since Ronald first encountered supplemental testosterone, all his indications for heart disease have altered favorably. His cholesterol has dropped from 243 to 207, his heart-protective HDL cholesterol has risen from 41 to 55, his blood pressure remains under control with smaller amounts of blood pressure medication, his scores on stress tests have improved significantly, and, most important, Ronald K. hasn't had a chest pain or a TIA in more than three years. If he makes it to ninety, no one will be surprised, least of all his doctor (me).

Let's look at the vast medical literature that relates testosterone to your heart.

Medical Literature

Coronary heart disease is the leading cause of death in the U.S. and most other industrialized countries. Atherosclerosis, the accumulation of fatty deposits in artery walls, is the most common cause of coronary heart disease. These plaques, as the fatty deposits are called, grow over time, continuously narrowing the arterial passage until eventually a blood clot blocks the constricted passageway, and, *presto!*—you may be down for the count.

Plaque is actually formed within the arteries as a method of repairing damage to their walls, and, of course, the blood enzymes that cause clotting also have a beneficial purpose, for they slow our rate of bleeding if we suffer injuries. The system is quite effective—when you're young. With age, however, these protective devices, while still serving their protective functions, also become the source of cardiovascular disease, and medicine ends up searching for ways to minimize the influence of the body's own natural design. Thus, millions of people take aspirin because it impedes the ability of the blood to clot. This is testimony to the fact that they regard themselves as far more likely to die of a heart attack than to be killed in an automobile accident. If the opposite were true, no doctor would be prescribing a substance that increases your chances of bleeding to death following an injury.

The assumption about any substance such as testosterone that allows us to circumvent the scenario that leads to heart attacks and strokes is that somehow it aids us in minimizing one or more of the factors that narrow and harden the arteries, or that it helps in preventing the excessive formation of blood clots. The male hormone does exactly that for men. It's also clear that when testosterone levels are low, results can be predictably catastrophic.

Way back in 1976, when unfortunately very few medical scientists were looking, there were hints of that. In that year, Argentine researchers made a close study of twenty-three middle-aged men who had survived heart attacks. The men had high cholesterol and triglyceride levels. They also had significantly lower testosterone than men with healthy hearts. The five patients with the lowest testosterone had the most significant array of negative risk factors. This study was a prevision of the true face of testosterone.[11]

More recently, dozens of studies have appeared. The famous Caerphilly Heart Disease Study conducted in Wales on 2,512 men found that persons with prevalent heart disease had significantly lower testosterone levels. They also had higher insulin levels and had less of the heart protective HDL cholesterol, which most heart specialists consider a far more significant factor in your likelihood for suffering a heart attack than your total cholesterol.[12]

Here in America, research was done by Dr. Gerald Phillips and his associates at the Columbia University College of Physicians and Surgeons. Phillips wanted to determine whether the *degree* of coronary artery disease in men would correlate with testosterone. To do this, angiograms were conducted on fifty-five male patients who had experienced chest pain or abnormal stress tests. What Phillips found was that the lower the patients' testosterone levels, the greater the degree of heart disease as measured by narrowing of the coronary arteries. And the men with the healthier coronary arteries not only had less advanced coronary artery disease, they had lower levels of major risk factors: fibrinogen; plasminogen, the clot buster; and insulin. In addition, their heart-protective HDL was higher.[13] It was a powerful convergence of observed effects and mechanisms. The wheel turned.

Another international study comes from China, where doctors decided to *treat* cardiovascular disease with testosterone.

The Chinese researchers took sixty-two elderly males with an established pattern of chest pain (angina) and administered testosterone to half of them, while the rest consumed a placebo. After a two-week break, they switched the treatment for the groups.

The effects of treatment were dramatically clear. Of the patients receiving testosterone, 77 percent had marked relief from anginal pain, while only 6 percent of the patients in the placebo group showed improvement. *Echocardiography demonstrated that blood flow to the heart improved in 68.8 percent of those receiving testosterone!*[14]

To those of us treating patients in private practice with the male hormone, these results are hardly surprising. I see heart patients all the time who have improved both functionally and biochemically with the aid of testosterone.

Are these discoveries all new? Well, testosterone is still cutting-edge medicine, but it isn't new. Consider the lifetime work of Jens Moller, a Danish physician, who began treating one of the worst types of vascular diseases known to man—diabetic gangrene—more than twenty years ago. Moller's clinic used testosterone at doses five to ten times higher than normal to treat the extreme pathologic changes characteristic of this dreadful condition. The result was a slowing and, in many cases, complete reversal of the progression toward amputation common in diabetic gangrene. Naturally, the patients also enjoyed increased strength and mobility. Moller documented these changes by photography and published his results. Amazingly, he garnered more criticism than plaudits even though no other effective treatment for diabetic gangrene exists to date. And, outside Scandinavia, his work still awaits significant acceptance.[15]

As my father, a recently retired physician, used to tell me, "Physicians tend to be down on what they're not up on."

Where Does He Go From Here?

Carter T., a Philadelphia banker who had been coming to see me once a year or so since the early 1990s, was certainly an accident waiting to happen by the time I got his attention in the fall of 1996. I had been warning Carter for some time that his lab tests showed a worrisome pattern for a man with a family history of heart disease. He was only forty-nine, but when the latest batch of numbers came in, it was my job to state the obvious. If he continued on the path he was traveling, he'd better make sure never to stray too far from a well-equipped hospital emergency room. Sooner or later, he was going to need all the help the ER personnel could give him.

His cholesterol level, which had been 210 when I first started treating him, now stood at 335, almost one hundred points into the danger zone, as those things are conventionally reckoned. His triglycerides were a fairly astronomical 900. His blood sugar, at 192, showed he had become diabetic. His insulin levels were at 70—four times normal. His weight was 230 pounds—significantly overweight for a fellow of five-foot-nine. And his blood pressure—here truly was a deadly indicator—was 192/118. A normal, healthy blood pressure for a man his age would be approximately 120–130/70–80. I looked Carter in the eye and said, "This is a lethal pattern. You could have a heart attack or a stroke anytime now."

Carter had other symptoms also. He told me that he was constantly tired—by four o'clock in the afternoon utterly and completely exhausted. Although he still functioned sexually, his interest was declining. He noticed that he was constantly thirsty, an indicator of diabetes.

I decided to check Carter's testosterone. He measured 410 ng/dl—borderline low. After a thorough physical, a stress EKG test, and other tests to rule out other possible causes of his low testosterone, I implanted testosterone pellets in Carter's buttocks in January 1997, gave him antioxidant nutrients, and encouraged him to change his diet. Looking at his lab work five months later, I found extraordinary changes. Cholesterol had gone down to 235, and triglycerides stood at 357. His weight had fallen a little to 220. Carter's most attractive and important results were his blood pressure—still high at 160/100 but, at least, out of the extreme danger zone. His insulin was now down to a normal level of 15. And his blood sugar, which at 140 still indicated diabetes, was now closer to the borderline.

What I was seeing in Carter's case was the way in which virtually all the cardiovascular risk factors begin to fall with testosterone replacement. Carter's testosterone level had gone up to 767 ng/dl a month after his implant. When I asked him how he felt, he told me his energy level was much higher and his ability to concentrate and focus on his work had returned. Sexually, too, his interest had come back, along with some early morning erections.

Paying Attention to Insulin

One of Carter T.'s risk factors—his insulin level—deserves a bit of extra reflection. Most laypeople are still stuck back in the days of cholesterol. For them, if their cholesterol levels are high, it's heart attack city, and if their cholesterol levels are low, all's right with the world. But, in the actual world of medical research, cholesterol, though still a significant risk factor, has been over-taken by many equally, or perhaps more, significant pointers. (For some insight into the declining fortunes of the cholesterol theory, see the sidebar on pages 93 to 94.)

Some scientists now believe that insulin may be an absolutely central component in the typical process by which healthy young people pass gradually—decade by decade—into the threatening land of heart attacks or strokes. You no doubt know of insulin as the pancreatic hormone that diabetics either cannot produce or have trouble using. Insulin is a substance that we absolutely can-not live without. It allows us to transport into our cells the glu-cose that we produce by eating.

However, it is a normal characteristic of aging that the body becomes less efficient at using insulin and that more and more of it gets manufactured to do the same work less and less well. This has a range of results, many of which appear to be damag-ing to cardiovascular function.

For instance, higher insulin levels tend to

❑ Cause weight gain—especially upper-body obesity.
❑ Increase cholesterol production in the liver.
❑ Increase the production of stress hormones, which by a reverse effect hinder the effectiveness of insulin.

The first two factors obviously increase heart attack risk. The third factor requires more explanation. When you eat, your body extracts glucose, protein, and fat from your food. Glucose, which is an immediate source of energy, needs to be regulated by other hormones, especially insulin. Insulin takes glucose out of the blood and stores it as a starch called glycogen. If it didn't do this, you would have too much glucose, or blood sugar, and you would be a diabetic. If insulin does too good a job, however, glucose levels become too low, and you can feel weak or even dizzy. Stress hormones such as adrenalin rush to the rescue. Partly by interfering with the effectiveness of insulin, partly by their own strenuous effects on the body, they raise glucose levels and produce a surge of energy.

However, as we get older, this system goes increasingly haywire. The body uses insulin less effectively—a state called insulin resistance—ultimately resulting in excess insulin production. The body also has less control over its stress hormones and tends to produce more of them quite independently of the demands of insulin. This stress hormone overload is partly the result of hormone decline. Testosterone has been shown to be an antagonist of the stress hormones: more testosterone, less stress hormone production. DHEA, another hormone that declines as we age, has also been shown to play an important part in controlling stress hormones.

Since insulin and the stress hormones compete with each other in many ways, greater production of one will result in greater production of the other, which may be why higher testosterone levels help to keep insulin down.

In many ways, testosterone and the stress hormones have directly opposing effects. Quite apart from their effect on insulin, stress hormones such as adrenalin and cortisol put enormous and, in the long run, damaging demands on the body. In effect, they stress us. Such hormones were well-suited to a day and age in which we tramped through the jungle, ever on the alert for the tiger's roar. Quick reactions and enormous bursts of physical energy sometimes saved us in those days from a fate worse than heart disease. Today, we're short on tigers, and most people are worn out by a steady diet of stress related to considerably less critical matters.

Stress hormones are major players in a process of tissue deconstruction that is a central aspect of aging. The way it works is like this.

In our youth, our bodies are protein-forming anabolic machines. To build up the towering structure of muscle and bone that was the youthful you, your body chiefly employed the powerful anabolic hormones, testosterone and human growth hormone, to take the amino acids present in the blood after digestion and turn them into protein, which is the very substance of life. So successful is the whole process that in our days of high and happy youth, it is difficult to harm us with anything less traumatic than a speeding bullet.

In the second half of life, however, the reverse process begins to take charge. This is catabolism, the breaking down of tissue. The stress hormones aid this process by turning protein back into amino acids and ultimately converting them to glucose for energy.

Although the body must use the stress hormones, almost by definition they lead us toward our downfall. Similarly, the anabolic hormones such as testosterone and growth hormone are life-enhancing by physiological definition.

Having made such a major fuss over insulin, let me indicate at last that the evidence to show that high testosterone is associated with lower levels of insulin is, by now, overwhelming. Dr. Elizabeth Barrett-Connor, one of the premier American epidemiologists, has collaborated on a study that demonstrates that testosterone decreases and insulin increases with each decade of life and that, independent of the age of the individual examined, there tends to be a direct relationship between the extent of testosterone decline and the extent of insulin increase. In other words, the more or less opposite curves that the two hormones make when graphed over time are not simply coincidentally related but apparently quite causally related.[16]

Cholesterol—Small Tree, Large Forest

Heart disease is devilishly complex, of course, and few physicians—certainly not I—would deny that cholesterol is one tree in the forest of risk factors. The question is: How big is that tree?

Ten or fifteen years ago, it was a redwood. Today it is beginning to look more and more like a New Jersey dwarf pine.

The fact is that, although everyone is told, "Cholesterol is very important, but you'll be safe if your level is below 200 mg/dl," actually the evidence for predicting future coronary events from cholesterol levels is poor indeed, except at the extremes. Certainly if your level is above 250 your risk does start to grow, and, if it's below 150, it is—unless you have other risk factors—very small. But the vast majority of us are between those two numbers, and, if we're within that middle range, where most heart attacks actually occur, cholesterol's capacity to predict whether you or I will or won't be stricken is practically nonexistent.

A quarter century ago, Dr. Kilmer McCully, a Harvard professor of pathology, described in children with a genetic defect the relationship between high homocysteine levels and lethal plaque formation in the arteries. He soon discovered that adults with high homocysteine levels were also gravely at risk for strokes and heart attacks, apparently far more likely to be struck down than people with high cholesterol levels. He published his results and found himself in the medical doghouse, where he resided for many years thereafter. He had cast doubt on the sacred cholesterol theory.[17]

McCully soon got some measure of revenge. As a pathologist, he performed regular autopsies, and he decided to check the relationship between cholesterol levels and observable arterial lesions. He and his colleagues evaluated 192 consecutive autopsies, ranking the severity of arterial lesions into four groups. These ranged from minimal lesions to severe, widespread atheromatous plaques. They then compared these findings with previously determined cholesterol levels. The average cholesterol was below 200 mg/dl in

(Continued on next page)

(Continued from previous page)
all groups. The difference between the people with virtually non-existent arterial damage and those whose arteries were savagely scarred by a wealth of lesions was only about 20 mg/dl—higher in the severe group. No doctor could possibly have predicted the difference on the basis of the cholesterol level.

Let me offer one final blow to your respect for cholesterol theory as currently practiced. Recent published results of treatment trials for cholesterol-lowering drugs have been severely discouraging. There was a consistent lack of benefit. True the drugs did lower cholesterol, but a bottom-line analysis revealed that, with the exception of one drug, there was no statistically significant reduction in the total number of heart attacks between the treated and untreated groups. Additionally, most studies show no improvement in overall mortality rates.

Moreover, the one drug that showed benefit showed consistent cardiac event reduction for all levels of cholesterol equally. This would seem to indicate that the drug had heart-protective effects but that those effects might well be unrelated to its ability to lower cholesterol.

I know that if you've been listening to the cholesterol gospel for decades now, it will take more than my brief stab at reason to unsettle you. But I simply had to get the thinking process started. Cholesterol has some significance; a whole host of other factors, including your testosterone level, are more important.

The Results

As a practicing physician, the important thing I notice is that testosterone's effects on heart disease are not purely theoretical. The hormone does what it's advertised to do. Patients come to me with chest pains, with indications of minor strokes, with wildly out-of-whack risk factors such as Carter T. had, and, once I find their testosterone levels are low—and I usually do—they receive hormonal treatment.

I wish I could say that every one of them becomes well and healthy and looks and acts twenty years younger. But medicine doesn't work that way. Most of us took a long time becoming old and sick. We don't solve our problems in a day, and some of them we never solve. Nevertheless, I would say that four out of five of my male cardiovascular patients show marked improvements when given testosterone. Many of them make extraordinary recoveries. They have shown me with unique force that, given the tools, the human body has the capacity to heal itself. Its own hormones are probably the most powerful disease-fighting agents on the planet.

CHAPTER 8:
The Complicated Prostate

The prostate has received a full measure of well-deserved publicity as a prime trouble spot in the male anatomy, especially in recent years. Back in 1985, most men probably didn't even know they had a prostate. Nowadays, nearly every man over the age of forty is all too aware of this little gland. They've heard that Bob Dole and General Norman Schwarzkopf had prostate cancer. They know that Telly Savalas; Steve Ross, the former CEO of Warner Brothers; and President Mitterand of France died of it. Perhaps they're aware Michael Milken is living with it. This cancer has become as dramatically associated with men as breast cancer is with women.

The prostate is, of course, a sensitive issue in the context of a book like this one, which proposes that many, if not most, aging men would be wise to consider testosterone replacement. Does testosterone accelerate prostatic problems? Certainly many physicians, as well as laymen, have been receiving the message that it does.

Yet, I think we're going to find that it does not. In fact, there's little doubt in my mind that a high normal testosterone level is one of the best guaranteers of prostatic health. I know for a fact that the records of physicians such as myself who have been active in the field of testosterone replacement strongly suggest such a conclusion. But we need to go further than merely anecdotal evidence, however widespread. We need to look closely at the medical logic that links testosterone in a thoroughly healthy way with your prostate gland.

You surely do want to take the prostate seriously, because its bad reputation is well deserved. At its best, this problem-prone little gland, tucked in above the genitals and beneath the bladder, inflicts a significant penalty—in the form of sometimes very severe urinary discomforts—on the vast majority of males who have made it to old age. At its worst, it's a site for cancer. Trailing only lung cancer, prostate cancer is the second most common fatal malignancy in American males. Upwards of 40,000 men will die of it this year.

You will sometimes find doctors who suggest that high testosterone levels are the cause of prostate cancer. There's very little evidence to back that up and much evidence to contradict it. Alternatively, it has been suggested that low testosterone levels might prevent prostate cancer. In a backhanded sort of way, there's some truth to that. We know that men who have been castrated before puberty apparently never show signs of prostate illness. This simply means that if your prostate remains a vestigial and unimportant organ, undeveloped and unused, it will probably never cause you any trouble. This may be true, but, since candidates for prepubertal castration are conspicuously rare, it's highly unlikely that this is the right approach to the problem.

For the readers of this book, the basic question must be, does possessing or restoring a healthy adult level of testosterone make you more liable to suffer either the annoyances of an enlarged prostate or the mortal terrors of a prostatic malignancy? There is certainly no evidence that it will. In fact, a recent study suggests that *low* testosterone is associated with increased prostatic cancer rates.[1] Could it be that the higher hormone signals program a message of cellular healthiness to the hormonally dependent gland? Let's explore the prostate.

What's Going On Down There?

The prostate is an unusual little gland, in some respects not a gland at all but an organ that contains about 70 percent glandular tissue and 30 percent fibromuscular tissue. The glandular portion secretes the liquid portion of semen, while the fibromuscular portion helps to open the bladder so that you can pass urine. The prostate is rather small, about the shape and size of a chestnut, and it's situated just beneath the bladder and above the rectum. In the average adult, it weighs between 20 and 30 grams, and it's encased in a thick fibrous capsule.

Until puberty, nothing much happens there. Then there's a growth spurt, and, in the teens, it increases in weight and doubles in size. A few fortunate men will have a prostate that never increases in size again. Most of us, however, will experience renewed prostate growth in our forties, fifties, and sixties. Urologists refer to this as benign prostatic hypertrophy (BPH).

BPH is benign only in the sense that it's nonmalignant. So far as we know, benign growth of the prostate has no relationship to the likelihood of cancer. The American Foundation for Urologic Disease estimates that more than half of all men fifty and above have enlarged prostates. Common symptoms of BPH include decreased force of urination, trouble initiating urination, dribbling (trouble shutting off the urine stream), and a feeling of bladder fullness even after urination. There can also be painful urination and a frequent need to urinate.

As BPH worsens, as it all too often does, more urine may be retained in the bladder, the above symptoms tend to intensify, and, in addition, there may be nocturia (waking up during the night to urinate) and incontinence. In a worst-case scenario, urinary blockage occurs and emergency surgery is necessary to restore urination. Not all these symptoms occur in most males, but a sufficient sampling of the worst symptoms occur so that it has been estimated that 10 percent of all American males will have prostate surgery at some point in their lives. And naturally, the odds for suffering severe BPH increase steadily with age.

The prostate causes all this botheration because of its position. The urethra, the flexible tube that transports urine from the bladder down to and through the penis, where it can be voided, passes directly through the center of the prostate; that portion of it is called the prostatic urethra. When a man urinates, the fibro-muscular portion of the prostate contracts, dilating the prostatic

---

Table 5: *Chart of Symptoms for BPH*

Increased frequency of urination

Difficulty initiating urination

Decreased force of urination

Reduced or feeble stream of urine

Urinary leakage (dribbling)

Feeling of bladder fullness even after urination

Painful urination

Need to get up and urinate during the night (nocturia)

Extreme need to urinate, sometimes resulting in incontinence

Urinary blockage, i.e., inability to urinate (a medical emergency)

urethra, thus allowing urine to flow from the bladder to the penis. In some men, as the prostate enlarges with age, it exerts undue pressure on the urethra, thereby obstructing the flow of urine and causing the diversely distressing symptomatology described previously.

A Bigger, Badder Wolf at the Door

Of course, if BPH was all the prostate could do to you, the gland would be only a moderate-sized blip on the medical radar screens. Unfortunately, your prostate can also kill you.

Prostate cancer is so common that when men over the age of eighty die of other causes and are autopsied, well over 30 percent of them are discovered to have had cancerous prostates, which neither they nor their physicians were aware of. But, in the majority of cases, prostatic cancer is so slow growing that most men not only never get sick from it, they never even find out they have it. It can easily take prostate cancer more than a decade to reach its detectable state and spread outside the gland itself—which is when it becomes dangerous. That's why when men in their seventies or eighties are found to have prostate cancer still contained within their prostate, most doctors recommend "watching and waiting" rather than going in for major surgery to remove the gland, which can be significantly risky in an older man.

The implication behind their advice is, "Look here, Joe, you're seventy-five. Why go under the knife when you'll probably be dead before this cancer kills you?" Of course, an exceptionally healthy seventy-five-year-old might think twice about that advice. Forty thousand deaths per year are ominous. And there are occasions in which prostatic cancer grows quickly. The likelihood that it will do so in any given man is usually determined by a biopsy of the tumor, graded according to an established scale called a Gleason score to determine how far advanced the cancer cells are and how aggressive they're likely to become. But such a predictive scale is only an approximation and is sometimes dead wrong.

Meanwhile, a major diagnostic advance has brought prostate cancer to the attention of millions of men who otherwise never would have thought about it. As it happens, the prostate gland, when it is bothered by either benign or malignant growth, produces a protein called prostate specific antigen (PSA) that can be measured in the blood. That measurement is called a PSA test, and it has been refined over the course of the past decade to a considerable degree of accuracy. Very young men will often have a PSA close to zero. As the prostate enlarges—even benignly—the PSA reading grows until a middle-aged man with BPH (even nonsymptomatic BPH) might easily register somewhere between 0 and 4 ng/dl. If his prostate is considerably enlarged, the figure could get quite a bit higher than that. In fact, using transurectal ultrasound to measure prostate size, doctors have worked out size to PSA ratios that give them a more precise sense of what's normal in a given individual. Men with very large prostate glands sometimes have surprisingly large PSAs without significant BPH and without prostatic cancer. It has also been found that approximately one out of five prostate cancers do not significantly raise PSA levels at least as long as they're contained within the prostatic capsule. For this reason, I always advise men over fifty who are having their prostate checked to have a DRE (Digital Rectal Exam), which involves the physician manually feeling the prostate to check for cancer.

As for the PSA level, doctors will generally assume that a number higher than 10 indicates a possibility that the problem is cancer rather than BPH. And a number higher than 20 is definitely a red flag for cancer risk. Further evaluation is usually suggested at 10 or above. Recently, PSA tests have been refined further with a "free" PSA test that appears to have a better capacity to predict whether high levels are due to prostatic enlargement or cancer.

Nevertheless, PSA tests are now a double-edged sword. Certainly many men are discovering and treating cancers that would otherwise have killed them. But, unfortunately, many more men are having their prostates removed—a procedure called a radical prostatectomy—and suffering the consequences, which, 50 percent of the time or more, include lifelong incontinence or impotence (and sometimes both)—when, if they hadn't taken a PSA test, they never would have discovered their prostate cancer and it never would have done anything to them. This is a cruel dilemma.

How Does Testosterone Figure in All This?

We know that the prostate gland is hormonally sensitive not only to testosterone, but also to estrogen and a number of other hormones. Now, if the vague popular opinion that the male hormone is dangerous to the prostate gland were true, what we would expect to find in the scientific literature is some indication that a man whose testosterone level is high is at a greater risk for prostate disorders than a man whose testosterone level is low. Let's look at this research.

One study, carried out by researchers at Johns Hopkins, followed the prostatic fortunes of more than fifty men, some of whom eventually developed prostate cancer or BPH and some of whom remained disease free. The study included lab reports on the men's levels of testosterone up to fifteen years before they developed (or failed to develop) disease. There was absolutely no connection between testosterone levels and development of illness.[2]

A couple of recent studies have also found no connection between testosterone levels and PSA levels. And, since PSA is the most reliable lab marker of prostate cancer risk, the absence of any relationship to testosterone is reassuring.[3]

These results are purely negative, but one Japanese and one American study measured a more intriguing possibility. Perhaps it is estrogen that puts the vulnerable prostate gland at greatest risk. As we saw in Chapter 5, estrogen increase is one of the defining characteristics of midlife in the male.

These two studies were both measuring the relationship to prostatic enlargement rather than cancer; nonetheless, the implications are intriguing. The Japanese study found that the men with least prostate enlargement had higher testosterone levels. Conversely, the men whose prostates were most enlarged had a higher level of estrogen. So striking was the relationship that the Japanese scientists concluded that estrogen levels are "highly correlated with prostate size and volume." The American study done on 320 New England men with BPH severe enough to be surgically treated and 320 men without BPH found that men with higher estrogen levels were more likely to develop BPH—and that if their testosterone levels were also low, their risk was even higher.[4]

What we are seeing here is the prostatic side of the theme we began discussing in Chapter 5—higher estrogen levels characteristic of male aging seem to put men at greater risk for illnesses of many kinds. The male body does not adapt well to high blood levels of estrogen—especially not in combination with declining levels of testosterone. And this problem of male aging may not simply be a result of natural metabolic changes in hormone conversion and in hormone excretion.

We have every reason to fear that we are becoming an estrogen-saturated society. A large percentage of the chemicals given to animals are estrogenic, many herbicides and pesticides produce an estrogenic effect, and many other chemicals that are at large in the land simulate the effects of estrogens and, in fact, are often referred to by scientists as xeno estrogens. Many of the most potent of these synthetic estrogens, such as diethylstilbesterol (DES), which was used for thirty years to fatten livestock, are now banned, but since, as one scientist put it, we live in "a virtual sea of estrogens," the bad effects are bound to continue. Not only must we fear the effects on the prostate and other parameters of male health, but the still-controversial subject of falling sperm counts in men may be related to estrogenic effects on the male fetus. Moreover, women are not immune. Some doctors have speculated that it is the artificial, chemical estrogens that are so omnipresent in our air, our food, and our soil that may be responsible for the apparently epidemic growth of breast cancer in women. In contrast to these are the natural phytoestrogens in foods like soy, which seem to have a beneficial effect on both men and women. (See the discussion of soy on page 192.)

If high estrogen does have a harmful effect on a man's prostate, can we speculate why? There are clues. As we saw in Chapter 4, every embryo starts off as structurally female, though, of course, in a radically undeveloped way. The release of testosterone sets the male half of the human race off on its own path of development, which will naturally include the creation of a prostate gland. However, within the center of the prostatic urethra there is a small indentation called a uticle. This is an early, undeveloped form of the uterus, and it retains some estrogen receptors. In fact, under the influence of an estrogen buildup, it can become inflamed and swollen and may even bleed. From this same area of the prostatic urethra there is also an outgrowth of cells that move into the body of the prostate and retain some estrogen receptors and an estrogenic program. High levels of estrogen can stimulate these cells to increase in size and number.

I am not, of course, suggesting that estrogen is the main causative factor in BPH. But it does appear to be the main overlooked factor. And, as we discussed in Chapter 5, estrogen is prone to increase in the midlife due to a wide variety of factors, most of which involve the conversion of testosterone to estrogen. You'll recall that alcohol use, impaired liver function, and zinc deficiency can all aggravate the process.

Zinc has always been touted for its positive effect on prostate function. This most likely stems from its inhibitory effects on aromatase, the testosterone-to-estrogen conversion enzyme. Indeed, zinc would appear to work hard at the process of inhibiting aromatase in the very neighborhood of the prostate. That little gland has the highest zinc level of any organ in the body.

It is also essential to say a word or two here about dihydrotestosterone (DHT), a more potent derivative of testosterone that performs many good activities in the body but which does appear to overstimulate the prostate at least some of the time. DHT is created from testosterone by the action of an enzyme called 5-alpha reductase. This enzyme is found in two types. Type one is found primarily in the skin, where it modifies sebucum secretion—stimulating oiliness and activating/deactivating hair growth. The appearance of secondary hair during puberty is a classic example of type one 5-alpha reductase activity. So is hair loss in men who are genetically disposed to it at a later stage of life.

Type two 5-alpha reductase is found mostly in the prostate, where it creates DHT from testosterone and, by doing so, apparently strengthens the fibromuscular portion of the gland. This is a useful effect so long as the DHT does not cause excessive enlargement. We know that sometimes, however, it apparently does exactly that. As a result, current therapy for BPH often involves drugs such as Proscar (finasteride), which aim to reduce DHT production. Such therapy results in atrophy of testosterone-sensitive cells in the stroma—the fibromuscular portion of the gland. Moreover, not only this area but the penis itself requires DHT for full activity. Consequently, complaints of impotence are frequent among Proscar users. It has also been noted that Proscar is only effective in treating the symptoms of BPH when the prostate gland is quite considerably enlarged. Your doctor should certainly keep this in mind, since in many cases symptoms of enlargement exist although the gland is only slightly enlarged. (And, startling though this seems, prostatic illness is so deeply unpredictable that there are many men with greatly enlarged prostates who show no symptoms.) Clearly, therefore, the only men for whom the side effects of Proscar should even be considered are those who have both symptoms and a greatly enlarged prostate gland.

It's interesting that one of the best alternative treatments for enlargement of the prostate is extracts of the saw palmetto berry (also called *serenoa repens*). Saw palmetto has been shown to naturally inhibit 5-alpha reductase, thereby lowering production of DHT. But since saw palmetto has never been associated with problems of virility, we must conclude that its suppression of dihydro-testosterone is more subtle and limited than that induced by the pharmaceutical approach. The herb appears to nudge the body into a window of roughly appropriate DHT levels, lowering them if they're too high but not lowering them so far as to create problems. All too frequently, Proscar lowers DHT so aggressively that it knocks the body out of that window.

There is also reason to believe that saw palmetto suppresses estrogen. If, as I've suggested, estrogen is one of the most significant factors in prostatic enlargement, then saw palmetto's surprisingly potent impact logically follows. It's interesting to me that in a study sponsored by Merck, the pharmaceutical giant, saw palmetto actually had more than twice as great an effect on increasing the urine flow rate in men with BPH as did Proscar.

I would say this isn't surprising. The drug, after all, has never been shown to have an estrogen-lowering effect.

Androgen Blockade

As you can see, *most current medical studies show a poor correlation between testosterone levels and prostate disease of any kind.* I believe those observations will be replicated in further research. The prostate is, of course, designed to receive an influx of testosterone; it has receptor cells specially made for that purpose. It is hardly likely to be coincidental that prostate disease of every kind occurs in the second half of life when sex hormone levels are declining.

However, once a man actually has prostate cancer, there is a form of treatment built around the restriction of testosterone. Usually this therapy is put into play when the cancer is too far advanced for the removal of the cancerous prostate to be at all likely to constitute a cure. The doctors, therefore, look for something that will cripple the cancer's ability to develop further. They have found that radically lowering the body's production of testosterone, a technique often called "androgen blockade," will set the cancer back, usually causing it to temporarily shrink and halting growth for a year or two.* Theories abound as to just why this approach is effective. I would suggest that androgen blockade constitutes not so much an attack upon the cancer as an attack upon the prostate itself. Deprived of the hormone that it needs for normal function and cell growth, the prostate sick-

---

*Restriction of testosterone—the so-called androgen blockade—is carried out in one of two ways. The patient may be given drugs such as flutamide, which blocks testosterone uptake by the tissues, or leuprolide, which resembles the body's own lutenizing hormone-releasing hormone and fools the hypothalamus into lowering its stimulation of further production of testosterone. A more complete and drastic reduction of testosterone can be implemented through castration (surgical removal of the testes). Unfortunately, as noted, with all these treatments improvement is temporary.

ens and many of the cancer cells that are not yet fully developed as cancer cells and which are temporarily dependent on a healthy prostate for their well-being cease to grow and may even die. This results in a temporary shrinkage of both the prostate gland and the malignancy it contains. Eventually only the most aggressive and fully developed cancer cells remain in the now shrunken and debilitated prostate, and, after the one- to two-year remission that the androgen blockade has provided, these cells resume their active and aggressive malignant growth.

Breast Cancer May Provide an Analogy and an Answer

In order to explain why testosterone is not only beneficial to prostate health but is far from being a substance that you should fear will stimulate the development of a prostate cancer, I want to suggest a slightly different way of looking at the relationship between sex hormones and certain types of cancer. Let's consider the other major hormonally sensitive cancer—breast cancer.

As you're probably aware, many women fear estrogen replacement therapy because they've heard it will increase their risk of breast cancer. If that were true, their fear would certainly be appropriate—after all, one out of nine women currently gets breast cancer in her lifetime. However, the breast cancer studies that have been conducted actually show relatively little relationship between estrogen replacement and risk of cancer—and many studies report no relationship at all. But even if it were ultimately determined that a woman taking estrogen puts herself at a small but significantly increased risk for breast cancer, there are other factors to be considered—factors that ought to mitigate tremendously any feeling that she was putting herself at risk.

First, there is the simple, statistically well-established fact that a woman on hormone replacement therapy is far more likely to live a long and healthy life. In the Kaiser Permanente study done in California, a paper published in 1996 found that the death rate from all causes was reduced by 44 percent in post-menopausal women who took estrogen.[5] In the light of this study and others like it, it is difficult to understand the reasoning of physicians who reject hormone replacement and who even argue that the menopause does not have a serious negative impact on women's health. The fact is that the loss of hormones—in both men and women—is part of the process by which nature leads us to old age and death.

Moreover, there is yet another very interesting side to the breast cancer question. When women who are on hormone replacement do get breast cancer, doctors have discovered that their death rate is markedly lower than it is among breast cancer sufferers who have never used hormones. This should certainly seem mysterious to proponents of the idea that hormones encourage cancer. But it makes perfect sense if we remember that organs such as the breast and prostate stay healthy in the presence of adequate levels of estrogen and testosterone respectively. They stay healthy because *appropriate* cellular activity is being stimulated by hormonal action. If breast cancers discovered in women on hormones are seldom as deadly as typical breast cancers, that's because of a characteristic of normal cells that we call *differentiation*.

Differentiation is the process by which cells that do not have any particular function are forged into useful metabolic citizens with different roles and tasks. For instance, as you would expect, the cells of your muscles are distinctly different from the cells of your intestinal tract. So also, the cells of a woman's breast have a distinct and characteristic differentiation that is nothing like the differentiation of the cells of her biceps or her heart.

When cancer occurs, the cells that become cancerous tend to lose differentiation. This is one of the most marked characteristics of any cancer—it takes over cells for its own purposes and, in so doing, robs them of their functional nature. The more advanced the cancer, the less like normal cells are the cells to which it has spread. Eventually the cancer cells lose all functional resemblance to other cells in the organ or tissue where they're found. Their very shape is altered; they are cellular monstrosities.

What has been found in postmenopausal women on estrogen replacement is that if they do contract breast cancer, their cancer cells are surprisingly differentiated, much closer to the normal type of breast cell than one would expect. As a result, the tumor is generally less advanced and tends not to grow as swiftly and aggressively as a normal cancer would. That this is what estrogen should have done to the breast is not really surprising, for the breast is designed to be healthy and functional in the presence of estrogen. Estrogen's role, after all, is to differentiate the cells so that they can serve their normal purpose.

What is true for the breast may well be true for the prostate. Normal concentrations of testosterone and its more powerful derivative, dihydro-testosterone (DHT), may well be harbingers of prostatic health not illness. Intriguing support for such a view is offered by several medical studies that show that patients with prostate cancer have lower levels of DHT than patients with normal prostates or with BPH.[6] The most recent of these, published in the *British Journal of Urology*, found, indeed, that the more advanced the cancer the lower the level of DHT. The researchers speculated that a low serum DHT in patients with malignantly transformed glands "may indicate a loss of biochemical differentiation of the tumor."

The Lessons of Experience

Although the exact relationship of testosterone to the risk of prostate cancer remains unclear, the experiences of physicians who have been treating men with testosterone for long periods of time is certainly extremely relevant.

Their records show astonishingly low rates of prostate cancer among their long-term patients—far less than would be normal in an average cross-section of the middle-aged and elderly male population. Dr. C.W. Lovell, whose technique of administering testosterone with subcutaneous pellets will be discussed in Chapter 13, has treated more than three hundred men with testosterone at his Louisiana clinic over a thirteen-year period and *has yet to see a single case of prostate cancer!*

In France, Dr. Georges Debled, one of the preeminent European clinicians employing testosterone therapeutically in aging men, also reports extremely low rates of prostate cancer in the two thousand men he has treated with testosterone over the past twenty years.

My own experience in treating men with testosterone replacement, although not yet as extensive as the two doctors just cited, is entirely reassuring when it comes to the hormone's effects on the prostate. In fact, I have seen a number of men whose symptoms of BPH have shown rapid improvement once their testosterone levels normalized upwards.

Sam B., for instance, was a sixty-six-year-old patient of mine with a long-term history of heart disease—including a quintiple bypass in the early 1980s. Sam, however, wanted me to help him with his declining sex function, his waning energy, and his persistent urinary problems. He had a smooth, diffusely enlarged prostate gland and a PSA that was normal for his age. His urinary problems were fairly standard for a man with BPH: hesitancy at starting urination, decreased flow, a need to urinate more frequently, and nocturia, i.e., a habit of getting up in the middle of the night to urinate.

I had put him on a saw palmetto formulation that did increase the flow and decrease the frequency somewhat. Real improvement came when I put him on testosterone in the fall of 1996. Sam took testosterone lozenges daily and, after a few weeks, he found that he was urinating less often and his muscle control was much better. He also had a lot of other pleasant surprises. As Sam puts it:

> *My sex life got a whole bunch better. Now sometimes I make love twice in one day. Lots of other things improved, too. I can tell that I'm stronger and have more stamina. My golf game is better, I can walk farther, I simply have more get up and go.*

Sam has always been an extremely physical person. He still goes hiking in the hills, hunts deer with a rifle and a bow, and gets out on the golf course two or three times a week in the fine weather. I wasn't at all surprised to hear how much improved he felt after taking testosterone. I certainly wasn't surprised to hear his prostatic symptoms were improving. Any physician who prescribes testosterone to older men gets used to hearing that story.

The prostate aspect of Sam's story has become so typical in my practice that it has led me to think that the real source of most prostatic illness may be hormonal decline and imbalance.

I would like to leave the reader, at this point, with one final thought, obvious but consistently overlooked. Benign prostatic hypertrophy and prostate cancer do not appear when a man's levels of testosterone are high—they almost invariably occur years after the initiation of testosterone decline, frequently thirty, forty, or fifty years after that decline has begun. Is it really plausible to assume that testosterone is the source of the problem?

CHAPTER 9:

Men, Women, and Bone

What if you were losing bone? I'm talking about the kind of bone loss that makes you wonder how many years are left before you become a cripple. That was the situation Tony R. faced. Tony had been asthmatic since his early teens. By the time he reached his thirties his breathing problems were overwhelming. More than once he nearly died and, as he admitted to me, more than once, "I wondered if I really would have cared." Tony was put on a massive dose of prednisone, a powerful steroid that, by suppressing the immune system, helps control autoimmune disorders like asthma.

On this new regimen, Tony's respiration improved, but, in the space of three years, he watched his height go down by an inch-and-a-half. His bone was being eaten away by his medication. If Tony had received nothing but conventional treatment, it would

115

have been an insoluble problem. Stop his medication and suffocate, or keep his medication and watch his spine dissolve.

I became involved with Tony's care in 1994. His medication could not be significantly reduced, but Tony could be given substances that help in the creation of bone. The most valuable of these was testosterone. In the last three years, Tony's height has stayed the same, and lab measurements seem to indicate stable bone mass.

Tony's case is doubtless special, but tens of millions of Americans suffer serious, crippling damage to their bone that leads many of them to the nursing home.

Why does bone loss occur? The real reasons are seldom discussed. There is, of course, always the possibility that bone loss occurs with age in both men and women largely because they're not taking care of their bones as they should. They don't get enough exercise or they don't eat correctly or they're taking drugs that damage their bones or their high-risk lifestyle includes lots of smoking and drinking.

I wouldn't want to suggest those factors aren't significant, but, in most people, the real engine driving the loss of bone mass and density as we age is hormonal depletion. A woman's hormone depletion at menopause is obvious, but she is also severely affected by hormonal losses that are very significant for men as well. And it is becoming more and more apparent that the most important aspect of that hormonal depletion in both men and women is androgenic. As we men grow older, we have less testosterone, less DHEA, and also less human growth hormone, and these hormones create the types of bone cells that build up bone. These are the hormones that draw calcium into your bones. In fact, these were the hormones that worked to build your bone when you were young and growing—in both sexes.

When does bone loss begin? The answer, which doctors will seldom give you, is that bone loss begins in your mid-thirties when androgen levels start to decline. No coincidence. Bone loss begins *because* androgen levels are on the decline. Bone is hormonally sensitive tissue.

An Evolving Plague

Osteoporosis, which literally means "porous bones," is one of the most expensive and debilitating diseases in America. Moreover, this condition is as common as discarded candy wrappers in an amusement park and a whole lot uglier. It robs people who ought to be enjoying vigorous retirements of the capacity to travel and lead active lives and enjoy their grandchildren and, eventually, even of the capacity to continue independent living.

Women fear osteoporosis more than men for reasons that will quickly become apparent, but any man who has aspirations to hang around until his eighties or nineties had better start putting a bone survival plan into place right now. Bone isn't lost all at once; it diminishes over a lifetime.

Many studies show that by their forties both men and women are losing bone at a rate of approximately 0.5 percent a year. For women, this is merely the calm before the storm. Their rate of bone loss can increase ten-fold after menopause. Many women have lost a third of their total bone mass before the age of sixty. One-half of all women have had an osteoporotic fracture by the age of seventy. For men, the storm comes later, but it has sunk many an aging ship. One-fifth of osteoporosis patients are men.

As the year 2000 approaches, the statistics-gatherers estimate that twenty-four million Americans have osteoporosis and ten billion dollars is being spent yearly treating it or dealing with its consequences.

Estrogen replacement therapy has attracted attention because of its favorable effects on the bones of postmenopausal women.

The effects are real, but, even in women, we need to look at all aspects of osteoporosis. For both sexes, that is going to include serious consideration of testosterone.

What Exactly Is the Plague?

Osteoporosis is a chronic degenerative bone disease that, over time, causes an excessive loss of bone. This results in a drastic weakening of the skeleton. The bones—especially in the spine, hips, and wrist—become susceptible to fractures.

People show the signs of osteoporosis in various subtle and not-so-subtle ways: low-back pain, diminished stature, hunched shoulders. Others have little indication that anything at all is happening until something breaks. Osteoporosis can be like termite infestation. Nobody knows its occurring until one of the hollowed out beams in the house comes crashing down.

No doubt when you were young, you thought your bone was permanent. It isn't—it's quite a fluid entity. So let's sing the bone loss blues. You're getting older. Just why are you losing bone?

The Bone Factory

Most of us have a highly inaccurate conception of bone. We imagine it as static, as unchanging as it is hard. But bone is active, living tissue, changing, developing, growing, eventually shrinking. It's only the dead bone of that skeleton hung up in one corner of an old-fashioned medical school classroom that doesn't change. Your living bone is a hyperactive city. Even as you sit quietly reading this book, it is being torn down and rebuilt. Each year about 25 percent of a typical bone in your body is dismantled—a process called resorption—and replaced.

In short, your bone, like the rest of you, is in the throes of transformation.

The remodeling of your bone is carried out by two specialized teams of cells. The osteoclasts are the cellular demolition crew. They're incessantly at work dissolving tiny areas of bone tissue so that the calcium it contains can be moved into the bloodstream. The reconstruction gang—known as the osteoblasts—are just as vigorously building new bone every day of your adult life, largely by depositing calcium phosphate on its protein framework. Osteoclasts vs. osteoblasts—it's the World Series of bone. If too many minerals are taken out without adequate replacement, bone density decreases—that's our termite analogy again. Over a long period of time bone mass decreases, and there is an actual reduction in the total amount of bone in the body. In very simplified terms, this is all that osteoporosis amounts to. So, by definition, if at seventy you have less bone than you had at thirty, the demolition team must have been working faster than the construction crew.

More Bone, Less Bone

At puberty there begins a dramatic increase in bone mass, a process that is set in motion by increases in the sex hormones, growth hormone, and the adrenal androgens. Boys in particular—fueled by the explosive onrush of testosterone—thicken their bone at great speed, especially in the neck, shoulders, and chest. That extra bone will serve them well throughout life, if it does nothing else than supporting the huge head that human beings are intellectually blessed with but anatomically cursed with. Overall, after the teen growth years, men have approximately 30 percent more bone mass then women.

With adulthood, the bones, of course, will never again significantly grow in length and thickness. In fact, the bone plates fuse and seal. Bone has reached maturity. In both males and females, it is at its maximum level of density and health in the twenties, and usually the first slight declines in bone mass occur around the mid-thirties.

Even before the firestorm of menopause, women are more at risk for bone loss. Their levels of testosterone are one-tenth that of the average male, and their level of DHEA, which at the cellular level is often converted to testosterone, is approximately 20 to 25 percent of the male norm.

Why Bone Loss?

Clearly the health of human bone requires a *balance* between bone deconstruction and construction. In youth, such a balance is commonplace and, as bone is dissolved (resorbed), a prompt and orderly replacement of its cellular constituents occurs. There is no mismatch between the activities of osteoclasts and osteoblasts.

Why, eventually, do the osteoclasts get the upper hand? This is still, to some extent, a mystery of aging. Yet what we now know suggests that a declining level of sex hormones in both men and women play a major role.

Part of the role they play is a permissive one. As testosterone and estrogen decline, they become less effective at inhibiting certain hormone-like substances called cytokines. The cytokines, especially one called interleukin-6 (IL-6), are extremely active stimulators of the cells of the bone marrow. That's where both osteoclasts and osteoblasts are produced, and when IL-6 levels go up, rapid increases in bone remodeling occur. Theoretically it isn't clear why this increased activity should affect the balance between osteoclast demolition and osteoblast rebuilding, but it is a matter of fact that the major changes that are actually seen are disproportionally high levels of osteoclast activity with consequent bone loss.

Some evidence suggests that our ability to produce osteoblasts is affected by age. Experts in bone development who studied osteoporosis in mice found that as the mice grew older the ability of their bone marrow to produce osteoblast precursors declined.

We know that the stromal cells of the marrow where osteoblasts are produced contain receptors for testosterone. And human growth hormone—also steadily in decline from one's thirties on—stimulates osteoblast proliferation and increases intestinal mineral and vitamin D absorption. It may be then that once low circulating levels of the sex hormones set in motion increased bone activity, which can no longer be supported by appropriate stimulation of osteoblasts. The happy balance of youth is now critically unbalanced due to hormone decline.

To counter this unfortunate situation, I believe that a significant percentage of men may need testosterone and possibly human growth hormone in quantities determined by measurements of their personal levels. More controversially, I think we are going to discover that women are going to benefit not only from replacing their estrogen, but, in many cases, from adding a small amount of testosterone to restore their natural levels. Estrogen will slow down the rate of osteoclast formation, but this only means that bone is lost more slowly. To actually halt, and perhaps even partially reverse, the loss of bone, increased levels of an osteoblastic stimulator is needed. That usually means either testosterone or human growth hormone, and, as you'll see in the chapter on human growth hormone, HGH (as it is generally abbreviated) is far more expensive than testosterone and essentially more experimental, since far fewer people have taken it.

Calcium is Critical

Your bone not only stands on its own; like most other things in the body, its ingredients are up for grabs when the body needs them. What the body particularly likes to take from bone is its principal constituent, calcium, which is a highly active mineral odd job man. Calcium is essential for nerve function, blood pressure regulation, muscle contraction, acid-base balance, and the excretion of waste materials in the urine.

Probably no mineral does more things. Although, at any given moment, 99 percent of the calcium in the body is stored in bone, the body will draw it out quite readily if, for instance, the pH of your blood becomes acidic. That can happen for all sorts of different reasons, such as lung and kidney disease. When there are kidney problems, acids are not excreted efficiently. In order to buffer the constant acid build-up, the body revs up parathyroid hormone and sends it to mobilize calcium from your bones.

Of course, there isn't any fundamental problem with this calcium extraction. It's essential and normal. And, when there is some temporary requirement for calcium, the bodies of young men and women handle the situation with ease. After the body has taken the calcium it requires from bone, HGH and the principal androgens scavenge around in the bloodstream for available calcium and put enough of it back in the bone to maintain that wonderful thing called homeostatis.

It's clear that protecting your bone will involve both having proper levels of dietary calcium (see the end of this chapter for suggestions) and proper levels of the hormones that know how to put that calcium where it will do the most good.

You Men!—The Bells of Osteoporosis Toll for Thee

The popular media may have given the impression that bone loss is purely a female problem. It isn't hard to understand why. Reaching adulthood with significantly less bone than men, women then experience at menopause a catastrophic 90 percent drop in their levels of estrogen. At much the same time, their supply of progesterone and testosterone radically declines, while their levels of DHEA and HGH continue on the downward slope that became established in their thirties. The bones of women become, in effect, defenseless before their enemies.

If we men are made complacent by our apparent superiority in bone, we are making a big mistake. It's true that the more dramatic effects of osteoporosis are going to attack us more slowly, but we are eventually in the firing line as well. One comprehensive study estimates that approximately 30 percent of the hip fractures worldwide occur in men.[1] Moreover, for reasons that aren't quite clear, when people over seventy-five suffer a hip fracture the mortality is sharply higher—30 percent—in men versus only 9 percent in women. The clock of bone loss is ticking for all of us.

Not one man in a thousand and very few doctors properly appreciate the relationship between the male hormone and healthy bone. Yet the facts have always been evident. Many studies have shown that young men with low levels of sex hormones (hypogonadism) suffer a reduction in bone mass and a premature tendency to bone fractures. A small study done two decades ago showed the first evidence of the fact that it is reversible. The researchers treated a thirty-year-old man who, by conventional reckoning, was just slightly hypogonadal (testosterone level of 374 ng/dl) but who was suffering from back pain and other indications that he might be in the early stages of osteoporosis. He was given testosterone. Within two weeks his back pain had ceased, and tests showed that his rate of bone mineralization had tripled.[2] Studies like this ought to have led to widespread investigation of the use of testosterone in the treatment of osteoporosis, but nothing of the kind occurred.

At the other end of the age spectrum, much current research has shown that older men whose testosterone is low are far more likely to suffer fractures as a result of decreased bone mineral density.[3] The American Association of Clinical Endocrinologists has estimated that among elderly hypogonadal male nursing home residents, two out of every three have suffered a hip fracture. At the opposite end of functioning, Dr. Daniel Rudman, who—as you'll see in Chapter 11 when we look at growth hormone—is legendary among hormone researchers, found that, in independent-living old men, serum testosterone levels were the strongest predictors of bone mineral density and total body bone mineral content of any lab variables he could devise. Old men who were anabolically rich were rich in bone as well.[4]

In my own practice, I have witnessed the consistent relationship between skeletal frailty and low testosterone in my older male patients with some astonishment. If you were to send me the lab reports on a seventy-year-old man with low testosterone before you sent me the patient, I would expect to find a man with low muscle strength and energy, declining or quiescent sexual function, and severely compromised bone density. I would almost never be disappointed in those sad expectations.

Androgen Against Arthritis

Arthritic patients consistently measure at significantly lower levels of testosterone than nonarthritic ones. And arthritis is, of course, itself a major contributor to bone loss. Three times more common in women than in men, it often strikes earlier and cripples more completely. Arthritis is an autoimmune disorder that causes your immune system to attack your joints under the mistaken impression that there's something foreign to you there. In a sense, therefore, its gender bias is not surprising. Women have significantly stronger immune systems than men.

Their life expectancies are longer in part because of that, but virtually all autoimmune diseases strike them with greater frequency.

Can testosterone be used in the treatment of arthritis? The answer would appear to be emphatically yes.

This possibility flickered before my eyes more than twenty years ago when I was enjoying the stimulating and varied experiences of a family physician. A vigorous, active woman named Carol Amwell, who had been trained as a concert pianist, came to see me. She was well along in the process of being crippled by rheumatoid arthritis. Her hands were grossly swollen, her knees and hips were degenerating. It looked as if she would become an invalid long before she was of an age to become a retiree, and I was soon at my wit's end. She was on all the standard treatments for her condition: gold shots, heavy doses of the corticosteroids, and sixteen aspirins a day. She grew worse. The effects of her medications as well as her arthritis resulted in her losing weight and growing continually weaker. It began to seem as if in another year or two the question might be not whether she could walk and function normally but whether she could survive.

Carol told me that she had heard of a doctor in New York who was treating rheumatoid arthritis with hormones. I encouraged her to investigate. The physician in question was a Canadian named Leifman, and he had established a clinic specializing in the treatment of arthritis with oral preparations of combined estrogen, testosterone, and prednisone. His treatment was clearly based on the idea that the anabolic effects of the estrogen and the testosterone would balance out the bone-depleting effects of the prednisone, which was, nonetheless, needed by Carol to dampen her overactive immune system and prevent it from further assaulting her joints.

Carol went on Dr. Leifman's therapy and began to experience a significant recovery. So much damage had been done that eventually she would require both knee and hip replacements, but her downhill course was altered, her energy returned, and she has enjoyed two good decades since then, fighting her disease to a standstill. I was impressed at the time and gradually started using the Leifman formula for other conditions requiring prednisone.

Since then I've introduced testosterone therapy to a significant number of my arthritic female patients and have typically seen measurable improvements.

Treat Inflammation but Beware Bone Loss

Corticosteroid drugs like prednisone are powerful anti-inflammatory agents that imitate the body's own natural corticosteroids. Their discovery in the 1950s was a powerful tool in controlling such inflammatory, autoimmune disorders as asthma, rheumatoid arthritis, and inflammatory bowel disease. I suppose every doctor has blessed their existence when they made it possible for him to relieve the terrible physical anguish associated with those conditions. But most of us have also cursed their side effects, which can include fluid retention, muscle weakness, obesity, thinning of skin, high blood sugar, loss of libido, and, perhaps most significantly, bone loss, vertebral fractures, and even necrosis of bone. Some studies seem to show that bone loss is particularly rapid during the first six months of therapy.

In men, the administration of corticosteroids decreases blood levels of testosterone and almost totally suppresses adrenal androgens such as DHEA—a testosterone precursor. Since testosterone is so crucial to proper bone balance, this may be a major factor in the osteoporosis-inducing effects of the anti-inflammatory drugs. The best approach so far seems to be to give corticosteroids at the lowest effective dose and to supplement with testosterone. Certain substances, such as calcitonin and bisphosphonates, which inhibit osteoclastic activity, may also be of therapeutic benefit. Obviously these are matters in which you'll need the careful guidance of an experienced physician. You'll want to make sure he considers the importance of testosterone and DHEA in winning the battle of the bone, so show him this chapter.

Construct Your Personal Bone Preservation Plan

In this section, I'd like to show you the essentials of a comprehensive bone plan. After all, a good bone preservation plan is as essential as a heart health plan or an anticancer plan. It would be poor value for your time, effort, and health care dollars to end up alive but in a wheelchair. Quality of life is probably even more important than extension of life.

We're going to discuss bone preservation under four headings: exercise, diet, nutritional supplementation, and hormone replacement. If your objective is the same as mine—to be able to dance at your own ninetieth birthday party—you won't want to leave out a single step in this bone preservation plan.

Exercise

In our comfort- and automobile-oriented society, lack of exercise is a major culprit. Bones develop by resisting the forces that act on them. Repeated application of physical stress to a bone will cause the bone to remodel itself and become stronger. Studies of athletes such as tennis players, who use one limb more vigorously than the other, have shown that one limb develops thicker bone. At the opposite end of activity, bedridden patients lose bone at an astonishing and frightening rate. Astronauts, though in the prime of youth and health, also lose bone rapidly because the condition of weightlessness does not offer the proper resistance essential for bone health.

So build an exercise plan into your life. At the very least, set aside half an hour a day for brisk walking. If you want to reach a higher level of bone, muscle, and aerobic fitness consider such activities as cross-country skiing, running, swimming, rowing, bicycling, or aerobic dancing. Virtually all exercise is good for your bone. You might want to take up tennis or golf. And, for stay-at-home types, be assured even gardening and housework is preferable to television watching. Your body thrives on physical activity. It was meant to move. Once you've increased your level of activity significantly, even if that simply means walking twenty blocks a day when you used to walk two, you'll notice after a few weeks or months that you feel better and that you've adapted to your new level of exercise.

It's also helpful to balance aerobic exercise with resistance exercise. This includes weightlifting and many forms of physical work. Resistance exercise stresses bone even more effectively than aerobic exercise, thus increasing osteoblast activity so that more calcium bone matrix is laid down. Exercise of all kinds, but particularly aerobic exercise, will reduce body fat and so minimize excess estrogen storage and conversion.

I won't tell you here about all the other diverse physical benefits you'll garner from your fresh-found exertions. I will only say that you'll be doing one of the best things you can do for the long-term survival of your bone. Because, without the pull and tug of muscle against bone, you're in for a shattering surprise somewhere in your foreseeable future.

Eat Right

Although in Chapter 13 I'll offer a few more extensive suggestions for a life-enhancing and life-extending diet, I can't resist pointing out here a few of the dietary pitfalls that every single bone in your vulnerable aging skeleton hopes you'll be wise enough to avoid. Perhaps the chief danger substances are sugar, salt, caffeine, and alcohol.

In spite of spirited efforts by the American food industry and its house nutritionists to convince you of sugar's harmlessness, it is—consumed in the quantities that twentieth-century

Americans regard as normal—almost certainly a health hazard. According to the most recent statistics, the average American consumes 139 pounds of refined sugar and high fructose corn syrup a year. Converted into caloric intake, that means that approximately one quarter of all the calories the average person swallows daily is some form of sugar. One hundred and fifty years ago, by contrast, the average intake of sugar was less than ten pounds a year.

Because so much of our diet is now sugar (and a whopping percentage also consists of the depleted refined grains marketed in modern bread products), we are getting insufficient quantities of folic acid, vitamin B_6, magnesium, copper, zinc, manganese, and other nutrients important to healthy bone. Our food basket is filled with empty calories. And not only do we come up short on important nutritional substances, but there is evidence that ingesting sugar depletes our bodies of calcium. In one study, sugar given to healthy adults caused a significant increase in the urinary excretion of calcium.[5] The effect that such losses have on bone is more or less immediate, since 99 percent of our total body calcium is in our bones.

Dr. John Yudkin, a British physician who studied sugar for more than thirty years, made another interesting discovery. He found that when volunteers ingested large amounts of sugar there was a significant increase in their blood cortisol levels.[6] Now cortisol is the body's own equivalent to drugs like prednisone, which we discussed earlier; it is the primary corticosteroid secreted by your adrenal glands. As you know from that previous discussion, excess levels of corticosteroids can cause osteoporosis. Bottom line: eating sugar not only displaces the healthier nutrients you ought to be consuming, but it enhances natural chemicals responsible for thinning bone. Bad news.

As for salt, almost everyone is aware that excessive amounts of it are consumed in the modern diet. Virtually everything in packaged food that isn't impregnated with sugar is doused with salt. Research has shown that a significant percentage of human beings increase their excretion of calcium when their salt intake climbs. As for caffeine—present in coffee, tea, and cola beverages—extensive studies of its relationship to bone loss have not been done, but short-term studies have shown that within a few hours after consumption calcium excretion increases markedly. Finally, although alcohol in moderation may not have an effect on bone loss, there is little doubt that in alcoholics it is very significantly associated with osteoporosis.

Two other aspects of diet that you'll want to consider are protein consumption and phosphorus intake. Many people do quite well healthwise on high protein diets, but too much protein can be a problem if you're confronted by osteoporosis. The body mobilizes calcium to buffer the breakdown products of protein, and this draws calcium from your bone. If—an unlikely event—all the other methods of averting osteoporosis explained in this chapter do not prove sufficient to protect you from continued bone loss, you may need to consider a low protein diet.

Phosphorus, found in many soft drinks, also appears to adversely affect bone health. Cola beverages, high in caffeine, sugar, and phosphorus, are simply one of the worst drinks around for anyone planning to protect his or her bones.

On the positive side, a healthy diet filled with a wide variety of fresh, unprocessed foods, including whole grains, fruits, and vegetables, is the right approach to protecting your bone.

Use Nutritional Supplements Wisely

For many decades American medicine adhered to the flawed notion that nutritional supplementation had little to offer people who were eating a healthy diet. Literally thousands of medical studies conducted over the course of the past two decades have demonstrated rather conclusively that this just isn't so. Vitamins and minerals can have dramatic effects even when added to the best diets. Therefore, a comprehensive plan for the prevention of bone loss should certainly include a careful program of supplementation.

Calcium. Calcium is, of course, one of the major constituents of bone. It alone cannot prevent osteoporosis because other substances are necessary to permit its proper absorption, but supplemental calcium is nonetheless an important and appropriate part of a bone preservation plan.

For postmenopausal women who are on hormone replacement, I usually recommend 250 to 500 mg of calcium daily. If not on hormone replacement, I recommend 750 to 1000 mg daily. For men who have evidence of bone loss I recommend 250 to 500 mg daily. There are many forms of calcium in the marketplace; I usually recommend calcium hydroxy apatite, a bone substance concentrate—however, make sure that the brand you buy assays levels of lead in the bone used. Most reputable brands now do this as a matter of course. As for dairy products, these are not the best or safest sources of calcium. Many people have a lactose intolerance that prevents their consuming milk, and excessive quantities of cheese is not a dietary recommendation I make to my patients. Clearly, you should not rely on dairy products as your main source of calcium.

Vitamin D. In some people, age and declining growth hormone levels contribute to declining vitamin D levels. Supplemental vitamin D(3) will be quite satisfactory for most people. Rocaltrol, the active vitamin D (1,25 dihydroxycalcitriol) is the best form of vitamin D, but it's quite expensive. I recommend it to people who have a medical condition that requires them to be on prednisone or other steroids.

Vitamin C. High doses of vitamin C (1,000 to 3,000 mg daily) increase the repair and replacement of all connective tissues. It also increases testosterone production; improves the P450 system, which eliminates excess estrogen; and helps provide the antioxidant protection that is so necessary as we age.

Vitamin K. You need vitamin K to manufacture osteocalcin, a bone protein that attracts calcium to bone tissue. Vitamin K deficiency impairs the ability to mineralize normal bone. I recommend 100 to 500 mcg daily.

Magnesium. Magnesium deficiency appears to be extremely common. A typical American diet contains even less than the Recommended Dietary Allowance (RDA), and most researchers believe that number (350 mg/day) to be too low to start with. As much as 50 percent of all the magnesium in the body is found in the bones. Evidence—particularly an Israeli study done in the 1980s—indicates that magnesium deficiency is associated with abnormal calcification of bone. This is alarming since the quality of bone may be just as important as the quantity.

A study conducted in 1990 by Guy Abraham, M.D., found that while women on estrogen replacement therapy alone increased their bone density slightly (0.7 percent), when a supplement containing 600 mg of magnesium oxide as well as other nutrients was added the bone density increased by 11 percent over eight to nine months. In the early postmenopausal period, women treated with neither hormones nor supplements typically lose 3 to 8 percent of their bone mass per year.

I recommend 200 to 600 mg of magnesium daily.

Manganese. The highest concentrations of manganese are in bone and in various endocrine glands, and evidence suggests that it is an essential nutrient for humans. Modern farming and food processing techniques have reduced the quantity of this mineral in the American diet. I recommend 5 to 20 mg daily.

Zinc. Zinc is particularly helpful in treating inflammatory arthritis and in managing the metabolic andropause in men as explained in Chapter 5. Take 50 mg daily.

Folic Acid. Folic acid helps to prevent the buildup of a compound called homocysteine, which is a triggering factor for osteoporosis as well as a risk factor for heart disease. Four-tenths of a milligram is the RDA. You should take at least that much but not more than 1 mg daily without additional vitamin B_{12} (1,000 to 2,000 mcg). Higher doses of folic acid should be used with a doctor's guidance.

Boron. Boron enhances the production of compounds related to bone health, including estrogen, testosterone, DHEA, and vitamin D. Take 1 to 3 mg daily. Very little osteoporosis is seen in parts of the world where boron levels in the soil are high.

Soy Protein. Soy is a valuable addition to the diet of both men and women. Not only does it block excessive estrogen, but it helps in the prevention of bone loss.

CHAPTER 10:

Testosterone
and Women

Although this book may bear the "male menopause" in its subtitle, I simply haven't been able to leave the other half of humanity out of the picture. I couldn't do it for both personal and scientific reasons. As a physician, I know this is important, vital, sometimes life-altering information that women ought to have.

As an impassioned student of testosterone, I also have a purely scientific reason for including this chapter: it makes no physiological sense to write a book on testosterone that shortchanges the female half of the human race. Testosterone can only be scientifically understood as a common human hormone with roles to play in all of us. So let's see what it does for women.

A few years ago, a very sweet woman, Elaine B., a retired schoolteacher whose husband runs one of the local clothing stores, came to see me because. . . . Well, I'm not sure why she came, except she had tried most of the doctors in the area and got no comfort. Elaine was fifty-eight, and for five or six years, since her menopause, she had been absolutely miserable. Her body felt sore, and her brain felt battered from a long battle with her nerves. Her sex life had shriveled, and her laugh—she has a very nice laugh—no longer rang through the house. She had retired at fifty-five, thinking that maybe with more time and less work all would improve. And nothing had.

Elaine had acute anxiety, periodically acute depression, and was subject to panic attacks. All her problems had started at her change of life. Why was that? I'm not sure her doctors asked, since her problems were mostly vaguely psychiatric. Elaine had tried out a wide variety of antianxiety and antidepressant drugs with little effect but plenty of side effects.

When I met Elaine, she summed matters up by saying, "I feel my life is totally out of control, and there's absolutely nothing I can do about it."

And yet, what seemed mental was, I believe, purely hormonal. As soon as Elaine switched from Provera, the synthetic progesterone she was on to natural progesterone and started applying a modest amount of testosterone cream daily, her "mental" problems vanished and her original talkative, bubbly personality emerged. Her sex drive came back, her energy soared.

Some of her depression had no doubt been due to the synthetic progesterone, which affects many women that way, but the other effects were almost certainly the result of putting androgens back into a body that was being totally deprived. Tests had shown that Elaine's ovaries were totally shut down, and her adrenal glands were producing virtually no DHEA or testosterone. Am I surprised she got her zest, her sparkle, and her libido back? Not a bit. Nor was I entirely surprised when Elaine told me a few months after her recovery that, in the worst part of her time of trouble, just before she came to see me, she had saved up a supply of medications so that she could kill herself if she didn't start improving.

The simple fact is one can't have a satisfactory life if one doesn't have satisfactory hormones. For women, of course, testosterone comes a little later on the scale of priorities. The first question is usually estrogen.

I sometimes ask my female patients the following question: Given an opportunity to try out a pill that will almost certainly rot your bones, dry up your vaginal tissues, make your breasts droop, suck the elasticity from your skin, double your chance for Alzheimer's disease, and double or triple the likelihood that sooner or later a heart attack will finish the story—all this in a single pill—will you take it?

No one, so far, has said yes. Yet, as I tell them, the decision not to replace estrogen postmenopausally is a decision, even if passive, to pop the body's very own all-natural aging pill—and it functions exactly the way I just described. What a pill that one is! Any woman who says, "I'd rather stick with nature," is certainly free to do so, but woe to her, if she underestimates the consequences.

I know you're expecting me to talk about testosterone now that I'm finally giving women their chance at bat, and I will. Nonetheless, first things first. The astonishing advantages of hormone replacement in women—replacement with estrogen and progesterone, that is—conditions everything else we say.

Nothing in medicine has been studied so intensively for so many years and through so many patient trials and investigations as estrogen replacement therapy. Nothing generates more controversy, phobic reactions, and confusion. Yet, surprisingly, it would be hard to find a treatment in which an amazing long-term success rate is combined with so few side effects.

We know now that the advantages of giving estrogen so far outweigh the risks that rational opposition to postmenopausal hormone replacement in women is very difficult to sustain.

The therapy's ability to offer women aging modification, disease prevention, and improved quality of life is so remarkable and has been so repeatedly replicated in medical studies that it's sometimes hard to know what all the controversy is about.

The average woman has almost forty years of life, from puberty to menopause, in which to enjoy the health-promoting benefits of estrogen. During that time she is remarkably resistant to aging changes and extremely difficult to destroy by illness. A young woman is simply the healthiest creature known to man. Heart attacks and strokes barely exist on the graph of a premenopausal woman's health risk chart, arthritis and "sore body" syndrome are rare, and immune system function is outstanding. Dramatic shifts to the negative are saved till after menopause. The acceleration toward catastrophe that then occurs in so many women's bodies is not coincidental in the slightest. It is hormonal to the core. Postmenopausally, a woman has lost the major programmer of her health. There is no dancing around the matter.

If you fear that estrogen contributes to breast cancer—and that is clearly one of the major reasons that only 20 percent of the postmenopausal women in America use estrogen—then look at the pie chart below.

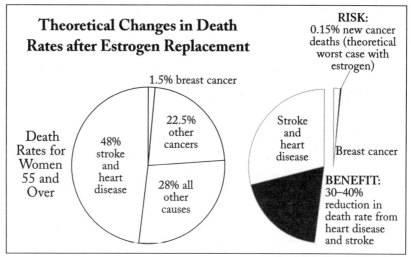

Theoretical Changes in Death Rates after Estrogen Replacement

RISK: 0.15% new cancer deaths (theoretical worst case with estrogen)

Death Rates for Women 55 and Over

1.5% breast cancer

48% stroke and heart disease

22.5% other cancers

28% all other causes

Stroke and heart disease

Breast cancer

BENEFIT: 30–40% reduction in death rate from heart disease and stroke

What that chart represents is the various causes of death for women in America over the age of fifty-five. As you can see, approximately 48 percent of all women die of cardiovascular disease, principally heart attacks and strokes. Twenty-four percent die of all forms of cancer—1.5 percent of the total being breast cancer. Another 28 percent die of miscellaneous causes, everything from automobile accidents to slipping in the bathtub. Hormone replacement is found in most studies to reduce the rate of death from cardiovascular disease by 30 to 40 percent—a drop in total mortality of approximately 14 to 19 percent. Meanwhile, worst case projections show an increase in breast cancer of 10 percent, which would represent a total mortality increase of .15 percent. The cost-benefit ratio turns out to be almost fantastically skewed in the direction of hormone replacement. The choice remains a very individual one for women, based upon their personal risk factors, but the meaning of these statistics seems very clear.

I'm sure you won't be surprised to learn that the *total* improvement in life expectancy when women remain on estrogen replacement is more than significant. A recent study supporting that view was conducted by Dr. Bruce Ettinger and published in 1996. Dr. Ettinger and his associates followed nearly five hundred women who belonged to the Kaiser Permanente health system in California. Two hundred and thirty-two of these women had been on estrogen replacement therapy for an average of seventeen years, and they were compared with 222 women who had been on estrogen for an average of less than one year during the same period. It was discovered that the death rate from all causes was lower by 44 percent in the women on estrogen.

I think we need to look closely at the reason why such a massive decline in mortality occurs in postmenopausal women on estrogen.

Table 6: *Benefits of Estrogen Replacement*

Reduced risk of heart disease

Reduced rates of bone loss

Reduced risk of Alzheimer's disease

Reduced risk of colon cancer

Reduced joint and muscle pain

Improved concentration

Improved memory

Improved mood

More energy

Better sleep

Reversal of vaginal atrophy

Maintenance of youthful skin quality

At the Heart of Things

Many women simply are not aware of the fact that heart disease is the biggest single killer of women as well as men. In fact, all the evidence we currently possess seems to show that if it weren't for the protection afforded them by their hormones, women would be significantly more at risk for heart attacks and strokes than their male counterparts. Men, after all, have significantly larger arteries, which take a lot longer to get totally blocked. Men apparently need that wider gauge because heart disease attacks them sooner, and the protection that testosterone gives them, although very great, certainly does not compare with the protection that the female hormones give to women. A famous series of autopsies done on dead American soldiers in Korea found significant evidence of atherosclerosis in those men. Their average age was only twenty-one.

Once postmenopausal women lose their hormonal protection, they demonstrate a startling and dismaying ability to overtake the other sex; in less than fifteen years, they're having heart attacks as fast as men. Which is fast work, indeed.

Yet, in women who replace estrogen, this change does not occur. Let's consider where this protection comes from.

Heart-Saving Hormone

The best estimates by reputable medical epidemiologists of estrogen's protective powers are simply stunning. One group of researchers reporting in the *New England Journal of Medicine* on 5,000 women on estrogen concluded, based on the improvements in their risk factors, that they would experience a reduction in their rate of heart disease of 42 percent.[1] British researchers, analyzing their own data, came up with a figure of 50 percent.[2]

It's not surprising, for there is hardly a single risk factor for heart disease in women that is not radically improved when a postmenopausal woman replaces estrogen.

Here's the lineup. Women who take estrogen have

❑ Higher levels of "good" HDL cholesterol
❑ Lower levels of "bad" LDL cholesterol
❑ Lower levels of fibrinogen
❑ Lower levels of plasminogen activator inhibitor (PAI-1)
❑ Lower levels of homocysteine
❑ Lower levels of insulin
❑ Lower levels of glucose
❑ Lower levels of lipoprotein(a)
❑ Increases in blood flow to all parts of the body including the brain, heart, muscles, skin, and bones

Let's review the meaning of these alterations in the cardiovascular milieu.

Cholesterol. As virtually every American is by now aware, cholesterol has something to do with heart disease. It's importance has been overstressed, but nonetheless, it is quite real. LDL cholesterol—the so-called "bad" cholesterol—only causes problems when it has been oxidized by free radicals, the process that antioxidant vitamins like C and E help to protect against. Once oxidized, however, LDL certainly is a bad player. Increased levels of it in the bloodstream trigger the activity of macrophages, large cells that engulf bacteria and various unwanted debris, including the particles of LDL cholesterol. The engorged macrophages then become foam cells, and these trigger changes in the wall of the artery leading to plaque formation. Plaque then fills up and eventually entirely blocks the artery, the whole process being called atherosclerosis. HDL cholesterol is called good cholesterol because it actually transports LDL out of the tissues and back to the liver for excretion. Estrogen's marked capacity to lower LDL cholesterol and raise HDL cholesterol must certainly be an important part of its cardiovascular protection.

Fibrinogen. This natural clot-forming substance in the bloodstream has been associated at high levels with a three- to five-fold increase in the atherogenicity of LDL cholesterol. High levels of fibrinogen make it far more likely that a blockage in a major artery will result in heart attack. Estrogen is clearly associated with lower fibrinogen levels.

PAI-1. Plasminogen activator inhibitor (PAI-1) decreases the body's ability to inhibit the formation of blood clots and so increases the likelihood that complete blockage of an artery will precipitate a heart attack. Estrogen clearly lowers levels of PAI-1.[3]

Homocysteine. Homocysteine is the newest buzz word in cardio-vascular circles. It derives from methionine, an essential amino acid that is present at fairly high levels in the American diet. Adequate quantities of vitamins B_6, B_{12}, and folic acid break down homocysteine, defusing its potential for harm. Estrogen helps to lower homocysteine levels and, in combination with vit-amin therapy, will almost certainly have a significant life-saving effect.

Insulin and glucose. Both insulin and glucose have been found—at higher than normal levels—to correlate strongly not only with risk of diabetes but with risk of heart disease. A rise in insulin levels is so common that many doctors regard it as almost a nor-mal, even if unfortunate, part of human aging. Estrogen's ten-dency to lower these risk factors may be highly significant in the overall cardiovascular protection it offers.

Lipoprotein(a). Levels of lipoprotein(a), a type of cholesterol that has a particularly high association with risk for heart attack, seem to be largely determined genetically, but, like testosterone, estrogen has turned out to be one of the few things that can effectively lower it.

Bone Preservation

Nearly as crucial to a woman's long-term survival as her heart is her bone. You'll remember how in Chapter 9, in the course of discussing testosterone's contribution to bone preservation, we also mentioned estrogen's role. It has been pretty clearly demon-strated that estrogen replacement therapy reduces the incidence of osteoporotic fractures by approximately 50 percent. Estrogen works by taming the osteoclasts—that is, it prevents the increase in bone resorption that occurs following the onset of menopause. Estrogen appears, however, to have no effect on increasing the rate of bone formation, which means it's important to set it in place as a sort of metabolic shield against osteoporosis before the ravages of bone loss occur.

In contrast to the effects of estrogen, a great deal of evidence now suggests that progesterone, its partner in the management of the female reproductive cycle, is a powerful bone-building hormone. In effect, this means that the two out of three postmenopausal women who still have an intact uterus—and who should be taking progesterone and estrogen to protect themselves from the greater risk of uterine cancer that estrogen replacement alone can cause—are actually lucky. The progesterone they take will not only negate (and, according to some studies, even reduce) any increased risk of cancer, it will add a powerful building block to their plan for bone preservation. A little further on in this chapter we'll get to the third piece of the puzzle: testosterone.

Estrogen for the Health of the Brain

We know now that women taking estrogen after menopause reduce their chances of getting cognitive impairments.
        —Dr. John Rowe, president of Mt. Sinai
        School of Medicine in New York

Since I can think of few life quality prospects more unappetizing than going into a mental decline as I age, I take the relationship between the major hormones and brain health very seriously indeed. In the last decade, scientists have learned how real that relationship is.

What catches the attention of most postmenopausal women is the fact that estrogen appears to have a particularly intimate connection with optimal brain function. And the lack of it is a negative of unpredictable but serious proportions. Like most doctors, I'm used to having women in their menopausal and postmenopausal years tell me that their memory isn't working as well, their concentration and mental sharpness lie under a fog. It's now clear that the vast majority of the time, these brain changes are hormonal.

This is why Anna Quindlen, a columnist for the *New York Times*, describing her own encounter with menopause wrote, "When I began to wake bolt upright in the middle of the night and started forgetting the names of my children, I initially thought I was losing my mind not simply my fertility." Naturally, being a trained reporter, she soon began learning the facts about hormones.

The truth is that, throughout your adult life, estrogen is hard at work in your brain supporting and provoking the densest possible web of dendrites and axons, the neuronal filaments, which, by connecting one brain cell to the next, facilitate communications and make possible an active, creative, memory-laden mind. Estrogen causes those brain cells to be more sensitive to nerve growth factor, a protein whose main function is to stimulate the growth of dendrites and axons.

Studies in rats have shown that when a female rat's ovaries are removed, her neuronal filaments begin to retract, and the dense web of interconnections is thinned out. If we assume the same effects in humans then the observed actions of postmenopausal estrogen deprivation would be, to a significant degree, explained.

Moreover, a fall in estrogen triggers a decrease in blood flow to all parts of the body including the brain, heart, muscles, skin, and bone. Brain scans of the vascular system of the brain have showed increased circulation when estrogen is added. That means as well that there must be an increase in the delivery of oxygen and essential nutrients. It's difficult to overemphasize how important it is to keep the highways open.

A final and perhaps most critical point refers to enzymatic changes. Dr. Bruce McEwen, a neurobiologist at Rockefeller University in New York, has shown estrogen spurs the production of choline acetyltransferase, a major enzyme in the brain that is needed to synthesize acetylcholine.[4] Acetylcholine is one of the brain's primary neurotransmitters, a substance that makes possible the final transmission of messages from one brain cell to the next.

People afflicted with Alzheimer's disease—the most damaging and irreversible of the dementias—have levels of choline acetyltransferase 60 to 90 percent below the human norm. That could be caused by a shortage of estrogen, which brings us back to the very large question: is there a connection between estrogen and Alzheimer's?

At this stage of investigation, the clear answer is probably. Indeed, many scientists would now say that we even know why a woman is far more likely to develop Alzheimer's than a man. Paradoxically, the answer appears to be a female shortage of the female hormone. Approximately 80 percent of a woman's estrogen is lost during menopause. There is no comparable male decline.

"Now, just hold on, Dr. Shippen," I hear you muttering, "surely postmenopausal women don't have even less estrogen than men?" When it comes to the brain, they do, because of the mechanism you're already familar with—aromatase conversion. The brain is so richly supplied with the aromatase enzyme that by conversion from testosterone, a man's brain is kept richly saturated with estrogen, in sharp contrast with the relative estrogen deprivation a woman's brain experiences once her ovaries have shut down. Of course, on the male side, this depends on maintenance of adequate testosterone. When testosterone levels in elderly men decline too steeply, either because of natural changes or because of medical treatment that blocks testosterone, brain function begins to slide downhill quite quickly. I've seen this occur with alarming consistency.

If estrogen protects brain function, will administering it to a postmenopausal woman prevent Alzheimer's? The answer appears to be yes. Researchers at the University of Southern California were curious about that very question. They studied 235 older women. Eighteen percent of those who had not had estrogen therapy were eventually diagnosed with Alzheimer's disease, compared with only 7 percent of the women who had received postmenopausal estrogen replacement therapy. In other words, the women on estrogen were less than half as likely to develop Alzheimer's.[5]

Even more striking because of its larger size was a study conducted by Dr. Victor Henderson of the University of Southern California. He and his associates examined the death certificates and the medical charts of 2,529 women who had lived in Leisure World retirement communities in southern California and had died between 1981 and 1992. Dr. Henderson discovered that the women who had been on hormone replacement had been 40 percent less likely to develop Alzheimer's disease. Moreover, the protection increased with length of use. Women who had taken estrogen for more than seven years were 50 percent less at risk.[6]

Further studies—one as recent as last year conducted in New York City—have confirmed the pattern.[7] Since Alzheimer's disease is epidemic among the very old, it is astonishing to me that these effects have not been greeted with more extensive publicity. I speak to intelligent, well-informed female patients all the time who are not aware of the connection.

Moreover, even in perfectly healthy postmenopausal women, estrogen seems at the very least to be useful in supporting memory.

When doctors at Stanford University gave recall tests to seventy-two older women who were estrogen users (average duration of use: thirteen years) and a control group of seventy-two women of similar age and education who did not take the hormone, they discovered that the ability to remember names was 39 percent better among the hormone users. Dr. Barbara B. Sherwin, a professor of psychology at McGill University, did a similar study using a battery of neuropsychological tests and found that women taking estrogen performed comparatively better on tests of their verbal memory.[8]

As Dr. Frederick Naftolin, chairman of the department of obstetrics and gynecology at Yale University School of Medicine put it recently, "There is not a cell in the brain that is not estrogen-sensitive directly."

This may also explain the well-observed tendency of postmenopausal women to experience depression, even when that has never been a problem in their life before.

Consider Laura R., a fifty-three-year-old schoolteacher, who came to me in the late stages of menopause suffering from a small cluster of symptoms. Her heat flashes were horrendous, she found herself urinating constantly, sometimes several times an hour, and her bones and joints ached so much that she found herself taking six aspirins a day without satisfactory relief. What troubled Laura most, however, was the complete loss of energy and the gray cloud of depression that followed her everywhere. She had to watch that she didn't snap at the schoolchildren, she felt like a mean, grouchy person, and, to this irrational, hormonally induced depression, was added the more or less reasonable sense of depression created by her constant state of exhaustion. As Laura put it, "Every day felt like a day when one has only had three hours sleep."

I gave Laura a combination of estrogen, progesterone, and testosterone, and her recovery was surprisingly quick. She found that after two to three weeks, she felt about 80 percent recovered from all of her symptoms. The aches and pains were much better, her urination was under control, her energy was back almost to normal, and, as Laura put it, "My best friend tells me I smile a lot more."

Laura showed a fairly typical medley of menopausal symptoms, and there is nothing unusual about her recovery from them. The human body does not respond well to the loss of its supporting hormonal cast.

Certainly, the human brain does not. To date, the evidence seems overwhelming that estrogen stimulates brain function and offers substantial protection against the worst of brain diseases. By the age of eighty, one out of six women has contracted Alzheimer's. It appears that estrogen replacement therapy could cut that number by half.

Keep Your Skin On

A young woman's skin is a remarkably soft, smooth, and attractive surface, and I know for a fact—because countless women have told me so—that as women get older, specifically as they go through the menopause, they are genuinely concerned about maintaining those admirable surface qualities.

The wrinkling and coarsening of skin that generally occurs in the second half of life is largely the result of hormonal changes. Studies have shown that the condition of a woman's skin depends more on the age at which menopause occurs than on chronological age. In other words, it's how many years you've been without estrogen, rather than how old you are, that determines your skin age.

Estrogen has several important effects. The layer of subcutaneous fat under the epidermis that gives firmness and resilence to the skin remains nicely plumped out as long as a woman has sufficient estrogen.

Estrogen maintains moisture in the skin by enhancing the production of hyaluronic acid, a substance that keeps water in the tissues.

Finally, estrogen maintains the thickness of the skin by supporting the production of collagen, the connective tissue without which the structure and tone of the skin begins to collapse. When collagen production falls off as a result of estrogen deficiency, a woman's features rapidly begin to crumble and sag. The lack of collagen together with the loss of subcutaneous fat causes tissues to weaken, bruise at the slightest trauma or bump, tear with the removal of tape from a bandage. Researchers at Kings College Hospital in London have reported that skin in women nearing sixty who do not take estrogen is only half as thick as among those who do.

Enter Testosterone

It's clear to me that for most women estrogen replacement—if they choose it—will provide almost miraculous support for their health and fundamental sense of well being. So why would they want testosterone, too?

Well, first of all because there's at least one extremely important aspect of life that I didn't mention in the estrogen portion of this chapter: sex. The reason I didn't mention it is that, in both men and women, sexual feelings are most directly stimulated by testosterone.

According to one study, 86 percent of post-menopausal women report a decline in their libido and level of sexual activity.[9] Although some part of this change will be due to estrogenic deficiency resulting in vaginal atrophy, loss of energy, and increased depression, most of it is actually caused by a decline in androgens.

Overall, a woman's levels of testosterone decline by approximately 50 percent in the years after menopause. Perhaps half of this decline is due to the complete shutdown of testosterone production in the ovaries. Equally important, however, is declining production of two other important steroids, androstenedione and DHEA, in the adrenal glands. These two hormones have relatively weak androgenic action of their own, but by a convenient process they are converted to testosterone intracellularly throughout the body—peripheral conversion, as it's called.

In many women, testosterone levels begin falling even before menopause sometimes resulting in a declining level of sexual interest as early as the late thirties.

Most women are certainly not aware that the most sexual areas of their body are packed with testosterone receptors. When a girl reaches puberty, it is testosterone that stimulates the growth of pubic hair and underarm hair. At the same time, there are testosterone receptors in the nipples of her developing breasts and a heavy concentration in the area of her vagina and clitoris. Without testosterone flowing to those regions, no bells will ring, no birds will sing, and "turning on" is turned off.

By the time they reach their forties or fifties many women report a marked sexual decline, sometimes even a feeling of complete sexual deadness. Some of them wonder why estrogen replacement therapy doesn't bring back the feelings they used to know and love. Happily, testosterone does. I'm sure you remember the story of Janice D. in Chapter 2, who said testosterone had made her feel more womanly than she ever felt before. It's a normal experience.

Your main difficulty will probably be in getting a physician to even acknowledge that it's possible (much less, desirable) to

> **Table 7:** *Conditions That Lower*
> *Testosterone Levels in Women*
>
> Childbirth
> Chemotherapy
> Surgery (adrenal stress)
> Endometreosis
> Psychological trauma and depression
> Birth control pills
> Ovarectomy
> Normal aging, including menopause

check your testosterone levels. There is a great deal of resistance among physicians to the idea of giving women male hormones, and doctors are great at thinking up convincing reasons why they can't do something they don't want to do. You may need to show him this chapter. For a woman to have an optimal sex drive, testosterone levels need to be more or less in the range of 30 to 60 ng/dl.

Keep in mind also that testosterone's other effects also have a payoff in terms of sexuality. If a woman has improved muscle tone, more energy, and greater general vitality, this can only enhance her responsiveness once she begins to feel the first stirrings of resurrected sexuality.

Bone . . . Going, Going, Gone

For many, perhaps most, women there is no quality of life issue in their later years so crucial as the struggle to retain bone. One only has to look at the frail arms and shoulders of so many older women to realize that anything a woman can do to resist this holocaust of bone, she must do.

In spite of the favorable effects of estrogen and progesterone replacement, there's little doubt that testosterone can add a needed extra boost. Few women realize what a strong association the male hormone has with their bone health. One recent study showed that the lower a postmenopausal woman's testosterone levels were, the greater her loss of height—the height loss being a direct result of vertebral fractures of the spine.

This is only part of a general picture that increasingly shows androgens and estrogens as independent and additive determinants of bone density. Originally it was thought that estrogen regulated bone mass in women, while testosterone performed the same function in men. We now have studies showing that when women receive implants of estrogen plus testosterone, they show improved bone density over women receiving estrogen alone.[10]

The Solution to an Embarrassing Problem

One postmenopausal problem that women don't particularly want to talk about—except sometimes to their doctors—is a leaky bladder. Yet millions of women begin to suffer bladder leakage in their forties and fifties and don't know what to do about it. Most often they find that when they laugh, cough, or make some intense physical effort, urine escapes. As one patient put it, "Three sneezes, and it's time for a change of underwear."

The reason for the problem is loss of muscle tone in the muscles of the pelvic sling, the *levator ani*. Those of you who read Chapter 6 on male sexuality will remember how important this area is. In both men and women, these muscles are peculiarly dependent on testosterone. Women who have bladder leakage find that rubbing a small amount of testosterone cream into the area between the bottom of the vagina and the anus will strengthen those muscles especially if combined with Kegel exercises, an easy-to-do program that involves periodically contracting the muscles in the pelvic area. (See Appendix 2.) Kegel exercises also have a highly favorable effect on sexual function in women as well as men.

Are There "Masculinizing" Side Effects?

Excessive doses of testosterone can cause growth of facial hair and, in extreme cases, a deepening of the voice. Fundamentally, however, there is no justification for a woman ever taking doses high enough to cause such problems. Testosterone is a natural part of a woman's body, and the small supplemental replacement doses that a competent physician will prescribe will simply bring her back into her normal range—the place where she was from puberty to menopause; the period in which, in all probability, she felt at her physical best.

What a woman whose levels have been less than ideal is going to notice when she takes testosterone is a resurgence of energy, very possibly an improvement in muscle tone and relief from aches and pains, an improvement in bladder problems, and, in most cases, an improvement in sexual desire and energy.

Putting a Postmenopausal Treatment Plan in Place

Hormones are critical and have been proven to increase the quality of life. Affecting everything from mood and mental status to overt catastrophic disease patterns, their significance is no longer in doubt. Hormones accomplish their effects with one of the safest track records of any chronic treatments known to man or woman. If you survey physicians, you will find they report minimal side effects.

Their reports will be even more favorable, if they attempt to tailor their treatment to their patient. Not everyone goes downhill hormonally at the same speed or to the same extent. As in most other health matters, there is a fingerprint of individuality that marks every person off from every other. This means that the really competent physician will search for the "window of effect." He or she will work with the patient to discover the hormonal levels that are ideal for that person.

In women, this is bound to be somewhat more complicated than in men, since the average woman can benefit from the replacement of three different hormones after her menopause begins.

How a Woman Should Replace Testosterone

Not every postmenopausal woman is in need of testosterone replacement. Deciding which woman would benefit is done by analyzing two types of information: her testosterone levels as determined by blood tests and any symptoms and health problems that have occurred since menopause and that remain troublesome, in spite of estrogen and progesterone replacement therapy.

Women whose testosterone levels are from 10 to 100 ng/dl are recorded as being in the normal range. In point of fact, after menopause the real range is from 10 to 50 ng/dl.* I have usually found that a woman will not have an entirely satisfactory sex drive if her testosterone levels are lower than 30

---

*Occasionally a woman who has not yet reached the menopause is a candidate for testosterone replacement, and she should realize that her testosterone levels will be higher the later in her cycle they're measured. It is usually best for her to have them measured about midway through her cycle in order to best approximate an average result.

ng/dl. Moreover, in women as in men, an official lab verdict of "normal" cannot be taken as final. A healthy normal, as opposed to a nonindividualized lab normal, is what works for a particular woman's body.

If a woman finds that her libido is significantly lower than it was in the past, that her energy is down, that she has no spark and sparkle, then, in all probability, something is hormonally amiss. Those are typical symptoms of androgen deprivation. Loss of muscle mass and any indications of osteoporosis would also be indicators.

If you and your doctor agree that you should take testosterone, there are several excellent delivery systems.

The easiest is a cream or gel applied to various parts of the body five times weekly. Each gram of the cream should contain from 3 to 6 milligrams of testosterone. A very small amount of the cream can be applied two to three times a week to the external genitalia to stimulate sexual response.

Women with leaky bladders will find that a milder testosterone formulation—.25 to .5 milligrams of testosterone to each gram of cream—can be applied intravaginally with a vaginal applicator. It works wonders.

Finally, some women who find that testosterone is definitely part of the hormonal solution they've been looking for may wish to have pellets inserted in their buttocks for a slow, steady time release, lasting four to six months.

I hope that those of you who are in need of testosterone supplements will be lucky enough to discover that the male hormone is for women, too.

CHAPTER 11:

The Power of
Growth Hormone

Late in the summer of 1996, Gerald A. came to my office for a checkup and a shot. He's a nice fellow, who I've known for more than a decade; semiretired, but still travels around the state selling jewelry. It's his hobby and his vocation, as well as a continuing part of his livelihood. On this visit, I wondered how many times I'd see Gerald again. He had been suffering from the complications of asthma and emphysema for many years. He was seventy-two, and for several years had been taking part in a cardiac-pulmonary rehabilitation program to help maintain his fitness.

However, I was well aware that the last twelve months had been hard on him. First off, Gerald had been diagnosed with prostate cancer and treated with external beam radiation. Apparently, the therapy had been successful. But while he was out on the West coast visiting his children, a series of respiratory infections had battered his fragile lungs. I spoke to him on the phone after he came back, and he told me he didn't really feel he could cut the mustard anymore. I urged him to come in for a checkup.

I'm not sure what I expected to see, but, when Gerald arrived, one of my nurses called me out front immediately even though I was in consultation with a patient. I saw a man who was quite visibly on his last legs. Half sitting, half sprawling on a couch in my waiting room, Gerald was gasping for air, and his lips were blue. He had just made the supreme effort of driving five minutes from his home to my office and walking twenty feet from the parking lot into my reception area.

I had to administer oxygen to Gerald before examining him. It was obvious that his respiratory system and his vital energies were so compromised that his long-term survival was at risk. I didn't think his prospects for making it through the winter were good. His first bad cold might well be his last.

I did a series of lab tests and found that Gerald was low in both testosterone and IGF-1, the lab indicator for human growth hormone (HGH). If it weren't for his recent showdown with prostatic cancer, I would have put Gerald on testosterone because of my extensive experience with its positive effects. But things appeared to be quiet in his prostate right now, and I certainly preferred to let sleeping dogs lie.

The other possibility was human growth hormone, an important anabolic agent with which, at the time, I hadn't had much experience. I did know, however, that its potential side-effects were relatively minor compared to the benefits it might have for a patient like Gerald. And I had seen reports that a number of physicians were using HGH to treat people with chronic advanced lung conditions.

It sounds unprofessional, but the flat-out truth was, Gerald had very little to lose. We started him on human growth hormone that September.

It took about two months for Gerald to tell me he was beginning to have more energy. Good sign, I told him, and privately wondered if I'd be seeing him in the spring. Well, I not only saw him, but a lot of other people saw him, too. Hormone replacement gave Gerald sufficient energy and improved lung capacity to resume his career as a traveling salesman. The man who barely made it to my office alive now goes off on two- and three-hour car trips and carries his sample cases in to his customers. Gerald won't be running any marathons, but he has made one of the most astonishing recoveries I've seen in my twenty-five years in medicine. Certainly he has serious lung problems still, but he's leading a happy, fully functional life and may go on doing so for many years.

This was my first indication that all the hoopla about the anti-aging benefits of human growth hormone might have something concrete behind it. The noise had started in 1990.

One Study

In that year, a team of researchers at the University of Wisconsin led by Dr. Daniel Rudman published a paper in the *New England Journal of Medicine* titled, "Effects of Human Growth Hormone in Men Over Sixty Years Old." The study seemed to show that older men who took supplemental growth hormone gained lean muscle mass, lost fat, and looked and acted younger. The newspapers got hold of the story and there was a fair amount of media noise. And then it was quietly forgotten.[1]

But not by doctors and scientists specializing in gerontology. No one had really been expecting HGH to have these effects. No doubt its very name created confusion even among trained scientists. Growth hormone is essential if children are to grow to a normal height. Without it, they are dwarfs. But what does the hormone do for adults who have reached their full height and will never grow again? It turns out that human growth hormone is the body's most essential maintenance and repair hormone; that, like testosterone, it has major anabolic, muscle-building effects; and that when levels of the hormone are lower than normal, this inevitably leads to weakness and eventual debilitation. European studies show that adults whose production of HGH has been minimalized or totally shut down as a consequence of pituitary surgery do not, on average, survive more than ten years.

Rudman's study was remarkable because it demonstrated that normal older adults whose HGH levels had been decreased by age but who were by no means substandard for their years would show very positive effects if given the hormone.

As we've all noticed, people's body shape changes with the years. Generally speaking, together with increased fat, there's decreased muscle, thinner, more fragile bones, and thinner skin. Internally, there's also shrinkage and decreasing functionality of major organs. Most of these changes occur after the age of forty, which is just when most of the hormones, including HGH, begin to taper off sharply. An average woman's body is 35 percent fat at age thirty and 53 percent by the time she's eighty. Similar changes occur in men.

Combined with muscle loss, this growth of fat is, of course, a vivid illustration of the anabolic (building up) and catabolic (breaking down) processes that I discussed in Chapter 7.

What Daniel Rudman and his associates did was to take twenty-one healthy men from sixty-one to eighty-one years of age and divide them into two groups. Twelve men received three injections of growth hormone every week for six months and the other nine received no treatment. All the men remained healthy, but, by the end of the study, the differences between them were startling. The twelve men on HGH increased the amount of muscle on their bodies by 8.8 percent and decreased their total amount of fat by 14.4 percent. Their skin thickness increased 7.1 percent and their vertebral bone density 1.6 percent. The untreated men showed no significant changes.

Moreover, the two groups of men had begun to diverge in actual physical appearance. Stripped to a bathing suit, the treated men looked—at least from the neck down—five to ten years younger than they had six months before. They were now harder, leaner specimens. No physical conditioning had been required for this transformation. Hormones had been enough.

When Rudman's results were published in July 1990, there was considerable turmoil and some skepticism in the medical establishment. In the years since, however, more than a dozen follow-up studies have demonstrated that the physical results reported by the University of Wisconsin were no fluke.

We now know that HGH will change body composition significantly in older people. We do need, of course, to find out what this means.

What Is Growth Hormone?

You recall that the pituitary gland is the master gland, locked away in the center of our brain, which sends out the command and control hormones for the body's entire endocrine system. The pituitary also makes a very different and unique contribution to the body's functioning. It manufactures human growth hormone. HGH is a small protein-like hormone (peptide) with a sequence of 191 amino acids. Chemically rather similar to insulin, it's secreted in very brief pulses during the early hours of sleep.

The body takes much of the HGH up into the liver and converts some of it into somatomedin-C, another small peptide hormone generally referred to as Insulin-Like Growth Factor-1, or IGF-1, for short. IGF-1 is responsible for some of the activity of growth hormone in the body. It is also far more stable than growth hormone and exists in the circulatory system for longer periods. For this reason, IGF-1 levels are what doctors actually measure when they want to estimate how much HGH an individual has.

In a young adult, 300 to 450 ng/ml (nanograms per millimeter) of IGF-1 is normal. As men and women reach middle-age and older, their levels invariably decline. Averaged out over a lifetime, these declines typically come to 10 to 15 percent a decade. The result is that in older folk, IGF-1 usually range from a high of 200 ng/ml down to as low as 30 ng/ml.

At minimum, HGH must be present throughout life at low maintenance levels if the body is to function at all adequately. Some of the areas requiring an adequate supply of growth hormone include: cell replacement; tissue repair; healing; bone strength; brain function; organ integrity; enzyme production; and integrity of hair, nails, and skin.

What such a list seems to suggest is that the radical decline in HGH production characteristic of old age might be in significant part responsible for the obvious loss of physical integrity that eventually occurs. Let's look at a few areas where HGH is beginning to be studied.

Your Beleaguered Aging Immune System

If there's one aspect of your metabolism that simply must function effectively to ensure your continued passage through the delights of this world, it's your immune system. The world is a perilous place, and the microbes and viruses and parasites that regard your body as a happy hunting ground are seldom at rest. They assault you daily, and yet, most of the time, you feel healthy, feisty, and very much above the weather. That's a testimony to the extraordinary power of your immune system. Most of the time you aren't even aware of the battles being fought on your behalf by your lymphocytes, phagocytes, and killer cells.

But the sad fact is that as we age, our immune system does, too. One of the indicators of that fact is the shrinking of our thymus gland, one of the major organs of the immune system. In childhood, this gland helps develop our immune system, its principal task being the creation of T-lymphocytes, the specialized cells that find helper cell lymphocytes and eliminate bacteria, viruses, and foreign matter from the body. In late childhood, the thymus is the size of a plum, but at puberty it begins to shrink, and by the time we reach old age it's no larger than a small raisin. Some of the functions of the thymus get transferred to other areas of the body—such as the lymph nodes and bone marrow—but there's still good reason for thinking that the atrophication of the thymus has a long-term relation to immune system decline. It's interesting also that, according to the statisticians, a human being is least likely to die at the age of twelve, when his or her thymus is in full flower.

But what if the thymus could be regenerated? We now have considerable evidence in animals and some indications in humans that HGH could cause it to do exactly that. Research in the 1980s on dogs showed that when growth hormone replacement was instituted, "the thymuses of growth hormone–treated dogs regenerated, resembling thymic tissue of young dogs."

In 1991 David Khansari and Thomas Gustad of North Dakota State University completed a long-term study on mice.[2] Taking fifty-two mice who had reached the age of senescence (approximately seventeen months), they divided them into two equal sized groups with one group receiving growth hormone for thirteen weeks. Most of the members of that group were still living after all the members of the control group had died.

Although the thymus gland was not measured (it is difficult to find in a mouse), the growth hormone-treated mice had T-cell counts comparable to those of young mice. And, presumably with the assistance of their newly empowered immune systems, they had passed beyond the normal limits of mouse longevity.

Growth hormone research has also been done on the human immune system. Scientists at the University of New Mexico School of Medicine took twelve older women in relatively good health but with low HGH levels and gave growth hormone to six of them for fourteen days. The level of natural killer cell activity in those six women increased by 20 percent.[3]

Keeping Your Brain

Most of the anti-aging hormones discussed in this book seem to have a very direct, positive effect on long-term mental function. It's fortunate that they do, since our aging population is suffering severely from aging brain. Current estimates are that fully one-third to one-half of eight-five-year-olds are at least in the early stages of Alzheimer's disease, making it a virtually epidemic medical problem in the elderly community. And, as you know, garden variety mental declines, i.e., short-term memory loss, diminished concentration, etc., are also common.

More and more evidence keeps tumbling in to show that the neurotrophic factors, such as nerve growth factor, that are needed to stimulate healthy brain activity require continuous hormonal support. One example is the salutary effect that estrogen has on the human brain, discussed fully in Chapter 10.

It's beginning to look as if human growth hormone will eventually prove to be one of these major hormonal triggers of brain health. Radioimmunassays and samples from spinal fluid have shown that HGH circulates in cerebrospinal fluid and apparently crosses the blood-brain barrier. It would be quite surprising if it didn't, since further research has demonstrated receptor sites for HGH in numerous parts of the brain including the hypothalamus, the pituitary, and the hippocampus, which is a portion of the brain that significantly controls cognitive functions and memory.

This could be one of the areas that HGH particularly stimulates since medical studies have shown that memory declines in growth hormone–deficient adults and that improvements in memory follow treatment. This has, of course, made HGH a source of hope for doctors who are treating Alzheimer's, a disease which generally first manifests itself by way of memory problems.

Dr. Chaovanee Aroonsakul, M.D., of the Alzheimer's and Parkinson's Disease Diagnostic and Treatment Center in Naperville, Illinois, has reported noticeable improvements after treatment with HGH in both these conditions as well as in patients suffering other forms of senile dementia.[4]

In a study of over three hundred patients, Dr. Aroonsakul reported consistently lower levels of HGH in patients with Parkinson's and multiple sclerosis, as well as stroke patients, and found a "profound deficiency" of HGH in Alzheimer's patients. Dr. Aroonsakul has reported some improvement in Alzheimer's patients after several years of continuous HGH therapy. She believes that HGH improves cerebral blood flow, revitalizes neuronal dendrites and axons, and enhances repair of protein in the brain, causing an increase in the formation of RNA and DNA.

Further Research Necessary

Growth hormone is certainly one of the body's most powerful and remarkable endocrine hormones, and it rivals testosterone in its capacity to rebuild muscle strength and energy. I believe HGH will be one of the miracle substances of the next millenium. What we need now is a continuing outpouring of fresh research to determine its capacities and limits and to define its side effects. There is a strong likelihood that someday many men will be taking both testosterone and HGH and enjoying a double benefit.

CHAPTER 12:

Medical Testing

To think about testosterone, to draw up plans for avoiding, reversing, and minimizing the male menopause is, of course, to think about the entire condition of your body. You can't take proper advantage of a sensible program of hormone adjustment unless you're preparing at the same time to fill in all the gaps in your health profile. Health is a holistic goal; hormonal health is simply one large, enormously significant facet of that bigger, greater whole.

But how does one think about one's health? Inevitably, since every human body is unique and mysterious, you and your physician are going to want to draw upon every aspect of medical reasoning and every scrap of available knowledge. You don't want to know how the average forty-five- or fifty-five- or sixty-five-year-old man is doing—you want to know how you're doing. Part of the quest for knowledge involves a wide variety of medical testing.

The most interesting part of that testing is hormonal testing. It's best to admit at the outset that the standard lab tests that nearly all physicians will require when they're giving you a complete physical often have a very low level of predictive worth. They will probably tell you whether you do or don't have overt disease, but the hidden problems, the borderline conditions, the elusive hints of catastrophes to come—these are very often missed. Sometimes, indeed, everything is missed. I am reminded of the old joke about the elderly party who came to his physician for a complete physical was granted a clean bill of health and collapsed with a fatal coronary right outside the office door. "Quick," said the doctor to his nurse, "turn him around, so people will think he was coming in."

Nevertheless, I, like every other physician, give a full battery of standard tests and extract what information I can from them. I know, however, that hormonal tests offer a more illuminating window into the future. The pattern of hormone change is integrally linked with physical and biochemical shifts that forecast the arrival of common disorders. Moreover, as you've seen over and over already, the correction of hormonal deficiency averts or reverses disease states common in aging men.

What you'll need, if you plan to get back some of your youth and hold onto every scrap of your health, is a physician who believes in the value of hormone testing and treatment and who is willing to work with you to determine your present physical status. He will perform a physical examination and obtain a personal and family medical history. He will want to know whether you have ever had any serious illnesses, whether there is a history in your family of the early onset of such conditions as coronary artery disease, diabetes, or prostate cancer. He is, after all, trying to obtain a picture of your individuality—your definite past and, very possibly, your predictable future.

After reviewing all your body systems, he will certainly inquire about whether you have had any physical changes in recent years. Fatigue? Weight gain? Sexual changes? What about mental/emotional changes? Depression? Loss of optimism, ambition, determination? Personally, I always feel out a patient's attitudes in these matters, especially if he has reached middle age.

Once these basics have been laid down, it's time to start doing blood work, getting some of those numbers we physicians are so fond of. Here are the kinds of lab tests that I would perform. I think it's appropriate to do the basic screening as early as your late twenties or early thirties, and you should continue to do it at least every five years thereafter until the age of fifty. After fifty, do it every two to three years depending on health and risk factors.

Phase I: Basic Screening

❑ Blood tests (complete blood count: red cells and white cells)

❑ Complete chemical profile of body functions including fasting blood sugar, kidney function, liver function, electrolytes, calcium

❑ Basic lipid profile, i.e., HDL and LDL cholesterol levels

❑ Thyroid (T4, TSH tests)

❑ Testosterone—both total and free testosterone (Women should have their levels measured three weeks into their menstrual cycle. After menopause, random testing is fine.)

❑ DHEAS—a standard test for measuring levels of the adrenal hormone, DHEA

❑ PSA—for men over fifty

Phase II: Special Tests for Special Problems

Cardiovascular High Risk Panel. These are tests designed for men who show any one of a number of indications that they might be at risk for heart disease or stroke. I think that once you reach the age of forty, you'd be well advised to have your doctor order these tests for you even if you're not in the high-risk group. It's much better to have too much information than not enough.

- ❑ Homocysteine
- ❑ Lipoprotein (a)
- ❑ Fibrinogen
- ❑ Insulin
- ❑ C-reactive protein
- ❑ Helicobacter Pylori antibodies

Hormone Panel. Any indication that your hormone levels might be low will require further tests. The significance of these tests will be explained in the next chapter when we discuss choice of treatment.

- ❑ Estradiol
- ❑ Prolactin
- ❑ FSH
- ❑ LH
- ❑ Cortisol
- ❑ IGF-1

Phase III: Tests Specific
for Individuals as Appropriate

- ❑ MRI of pituitary hypothalamism
- ❑ Prostate ultrasound
- ❑ Growth hormone stimulation tests
- ❑ Adrenal stimulation tests
- ❑ Chorionic gonadotrophin stimulation test
- ❑ Repeat testing of estrogen/testosterone levels to confirm changes
- ❑ Glucose tolerance test or two-hour post-prandial blood sugar

Drawing Conclusions Is
Harder Than Drawing Blood

Once the results of this potentially very large battery of tests is in, you and your physician should be able to concentrate on your hormonal profile. Whatever your age—whether you be in your thirties, forties, fifties, or sixties—your hormone levels are changing, by and large, in a downward direction. This is true of everyone, man or woman, lumberjack or librarian. The inexorable depletion of major endocrine hormones is one of the most indisputable facts of human aging.

How much, then, have your hormones fallen? This, unfortunately, is a question to which, almost certainly, you will not obtain an answer. Unless you had unusual medical problems when you were younger or had an unusually farsighted physician, no one will have taken blood levels of testosterone or any of your other major endocrine hormones when you were young. In other words, in the task of determining your present hormonal condition, you lack a baseline. You can compare your present testosterone level with the average level for men your age, but you can't do a comparison with yourself. You don't know where you've fallen from.

This is important because, in all honesty, the significance of your hormone levels is difficult to assess. Here are the reasons why:

❑ There are wide normal ranges.
❑ It is not easy to predict the accuracy of a single measurement since hormones are subject to daily cycles (the circadian rhythm), monthly cycles, seasonal variations, and short-term ups and downs in blood level resulting from pulsatile release.
❑ Hormone levels can be drastically affected by medications.
❑ Nutrition, stress, and illness will all effect hormonal output.
❑ Aging will decrease hormonal output, as we've noted, but though the level of decline in a large body of people is quite predictable, the rate at which testosterone, human growth hormone, or DHEA will decline in a given individual is deeply unpredictable.

I can see that I've virtually convinced you that hormone levels are so confusing they're practically useless. That really isn't so. To confine ourselves to testosterone for the moment, let me point out that what *is* useless is the standard doctrine according to which a man's testosterone level is within the normal range if it falls somewhere between 300 ng/dl and 1000 ng/dl.

Such a notion of normality is virtually meaningless, unless all you mean by it is that 90 percent of all men do, in fact, have testosterone levels within that range. But a meaningful medical notion of normal surely contains an implicit approval of the level found, a suggestion that when a man's testosterone is above the lower number and below the higher number, he can rest assured that he is basically on track. In other words, his health and vigor should be supported rather than adversely affected by his level— he's "normal."

If that is what doctors mean when they refer to normal testosterone levels, then they're flat-out wrong. Your own personal, "normal" level of testosterone probably *is* somewhere between 300 ng/dl and 1000 ng/dl, but no one can say where in that range it lies. You may be somewhat too low at 600 ng/dl, or you may be quite adequate at 450 ng/dl. By nature, you may be a high-testosterone male or a low-testosterone male, and, without those baseline levels taken in youth, which you almost certainly don't have, no one can tell for sure.

Let's just consider the case of two very different men. One is a high testosterone male who normally averaged between 800 ng/dl and 1000 ng/dl when he was healthy and young. Now he is fifty, and he has suffered a serious hormonal fall. His levels are now between 400 ng/dl and 500 ng/dl. This is a catastrophe, a 50 percent drop, and he feels every point of it. Now there comes along another individual who in the days when he was young and obstrepously healthy averaged 400 ng/dl to 500 ng/dl. He, too, has reached his fiftieth year, and his testosterone levels have also declined. They now average from 300 ng/dl to 400 ng/dl. The drop is relatively slight, and he notices little change in function. He still feels like a very healthy specimen.

It's relatively easy to make such an analysis. Unfortunately, in the real world, the physicians who are treating each of these men don't have the earlier numbers, the baseline youthful highs. All the physicians know is that one man has levels between 400 ng/dl and 500 ng/dl, while the other is between 300 ng/dl and 400 ng/dl. And surprisingly, the man with the lower level feels much better and reports far fewer symptoms of the gray zone of the male menopause.

Getting Your Money's Worth

You might fairly ask: what then is the purpose of taking testosterone levels? The purpose is twofold.

First, it helps provide yet another clue that you and your physician can use to interpret your physical and mental condition now. I mean that your testosterone level is one important clue among many. Basically it will have to be interpreted in the light of your symptoms.

Consider this hormonal truism. If a middle-aged man is full of mental drive and physical energy, has noticed no appreciable decline in sexual function, has neither symptoms nor lab results indicating a high risk of cardiovascular disease, then he clearly must have adequate levels of testosterone. Without such levels, he would feel lousy. If his testosterone level is 400 ng/dl, and the above description fits him, then 400 ng/dl is a good and healthy level for him. What if his testosterone is 200 ng/dl? I suppose, theoretically, the same statement could be made, but, as a matter of fact, in all the hundreds of testosterone levels I've taken from men middle-aged and older, I've never found an individual with a testosterone level that low who felt well.

Clearly detective work is required. So often, good medicine is precisely that. What if a middle-aged man's testosterone level stood at 800 ng/dl, but he had all the symptoms of the male menopause? A physician would have to look for other causes. Possibly extremely low levels of other hormones, possibly some disease state which was not at first apparent. In this case, the man's high testosterone would function as a very important clue. It would tell the wise physician that he should not regard the gray zone symptoms that he was observing as the normal signs of male menopause. Rather, he should be on his guard. Something else would clearly be at work here.

Thus, relatively high levels of testosterone in conjunction with symptoms are a clear warning to check for other possibilities. And relatively low levels of testosterone in conjunction with symptoms are a clear invitation to try any one of a wide variety of hormonal approaches. Not all of them involve replacing testosterone. The estrogen question is, of course, equally significant for men. If one of these approaches work, then some of your questions will be answered. If your hormones were out of balance or if your level of testosterone was low *for you*, then such gray zone changes as muscle weakness, lack of energy, and sexual decline will show signs of reversal after steps have been successfully taken to address the particular kind of imbalance you've been suffering from. Special problems such as erectile dysfunction may require special testing by a urologist if improvement is not sufficient in a reasonable amount of time.

Learning from Treatment

In the next chapter, we'll describe in detail the various hormonal approaches that work.

I think I have already implied the second reason that taking a man's testosterone levels in his middle years (and, of course, sooner, if you can) is so important. Having those numbers makes it possible to gauge the effects of hormonal therapy. When a physician sees how much an individual's testosterone levels go up—or how much his estrogen levels go down—and he compares these hormonal changes with the changes in energy, mood, sex drive, and/or symptoms of ill health that his patient reports to him, he has something to work with. Let's move on to the next chapter, where we'll discuss these kinds of decisions in more depth as we explore the different kinds of testosterone treatment.

CHAPTER 13:
Treatment Plan for Male Menopause

As you know, I don't regard testosterone *replacement* as, in any way, a necessary or inevitable answer to the male menopause.

Nonetheless, it's clear to me that most of us, if we're determined to live long and healthy lives, will need to take charge of our hormone levels as we get older. We can't simply trust chance and the whims of our aging flesh. Remember always that as hormones decline, you decline. If you're a man, your testosterone level is crucially important to nearly every aspect of your physical function. I think you should plan to normalize it at a youthful level—or, at least, at a level not too distant from what it was likely to have been in youth. For many of you, achieving such a goal won't require direct replacement of the hormone. For some of you, it will.

Yet, even if that plan sounds reasonable and conservative to you, it won't necessarily sound that way to your physician.

The biggest hurdle for many physicians is making the decision to initiate treatment or even simply to test for deficiencies. I am eternally puzzled by the number of medical professionals who still feel that decline in hormone status and the characteristics of aging related to it are natural phenomena that should not be tinkered with because of unknown "potential side-effects."

In my mind, the question should rather be: "What are the side effects of failure to diagnose or treat?" To anyone with eyes, nothing is more apparent than the side effects of *not* treating hormonal deficiency. If you're longing to see the ravages of hormonal decline, take a trip to the local nursing home. The widespread disability that you'll see around you there is an unspeakable price to pay. The mere contemplation of it leaves a scar upon the mind.

I truly believe that there are no side effects to preserving or replacing your own personal, normal hormonal status—there is only the return of healthy bodily functions. After all, isn't this smooth result true of all our traditionally replaced hormones, such as thyroid, cortisone, and insulin? I have never heard anyone offer an even partially coherent explanation for the view that testosterone, estrogen, and human growth hormone cannot be replaced with equal benefit. *The body does not work well with major depletion of its major hormonal substances!* This is basic medicine.

The only side-effects are those related to our inability to replace hormones as perfectly as our bodies do in the normal process of secreting them. That's why getting the body to make its own hormones at optimum levels is always the best way. It is only when deficiency is irreversible that hormone replacement is necessary.

My recommendation is simple—encourage your physician to work with you and explore the possibilities of hormone therapy as soon as the first indications of the male menopause begin darkening your life. Women, I strongly believe, should also seek out a professional who will discuss the pros and cons of initiating a postmenopausal hormone therapy suitable for them and will pursue the potential advantages of including a small amount of testosterone in the mix.

Since Chapter 10 discussed the best modes of testosterone treatment for women, the rest of this chapter will outline treatment protocols for men only.

Establish Your Health Baseline

In outlining testing, the previous chapter laid the groundwork for determining your physical condition and acting upon it. Don't hesitate to try to correct as many health problems as possible before embarking on your hormone therapy. You should take special care to determine the possibility of conditions such as diabetes and hypothyroidism, which would have significant effects on your hormone functioning.

If you're undergoing any sort of medical treatment, make a list of the drugs you're taking and compare them with the list in Appendix 3. Are there any troublemakers in your drug bag? Some of them may suppress aspects of hormone function as long as you continue to take them. If so, your doctor must find less interfering drugs for you or your prospects of launching a successful assault upon the male menopause will diminish sharply. And since low testosterone levels are intimately related to many disease processes, ask your doctor to consider the possibility that testosterone treatment may so improve your medical condition that you won't need to be taking drugs.

If you're to have any hope of beating back the sludge tide of the gray zone, you'll also need to recognize the interconnecting links between a healthy lifestyle and your hormonal status. In some cases, change in these areas is all that is needed to correct and rebalance the books. Getting some exercise to control obesity and stimulate your metabolism, changing diet and reinforcing that diet with nutritional supplements—these changes constitute the lowest measure of essential common sense, if you want to win. If you ignore those measures, the best your hormone improvements may bring you to is a state of mediocrity. If you abuse your body with drugs, alcohol, or cigarettes, you may not even make it that far. True quality of life, exceptional vitality, and enhanced longevity is seldom extended to the self-destructive.

Try Some Nutritional Winners

Before explaining the hormonal treatment plan that I outline to my patients, let's take a look at some of the vitamins, herbs, and other nutritional agents that can tune up your heart, your head, and, specifically, your endocrine system.

There are certain common elements in aging that virtually all of us suffer to one degree or another. The most pervasive is circulatory problems. Blood is not going to every portion of your body with the ease and completeness it once did. Even if you never suffer a heart attack or a stroke, even if you die at the age of 101 from the deleterious effects of eating too much peppermint candy, you will still have had your style more than a little cramped in the previous few decades by cardiovascular impairment of one kind or another.

Another near-universal adverse aging change is the slowing of at least some forms of mental dexterity. Though many of us will be fortunate to retain full mental competence and intellectual power into our eighties and nineties, we will, nonetheless, notice some slippage. Words that are harder to recall, short-term memories that we have a difficult time accessing and keeping, simple repetitive mental tasks that take us twenty minutes when they used to take us ten. Whole books are being and have been written on the reasons for such change. We discussed some aspects of the problem in Chapter 3.

Two factors are clear: circulation to the brain is generally not as good as we get older, and neurological changes occur within the brain, perhaps partly spurred by declining hormone levels.

We're fortunate that circulatory and neurological changes— probably the two most serious challenges we face as we get older—have proven to be open to the influence of a wide variety of nutritional agents. For instance, it is quite apparent now— with a wealth of scientific evidence—that the availability and use of such nutritional antioxidants as vitamins C and E, selenium, and the carotene group have done more for the health of Americans than the majority of the pharmaceuticals developed in the past three decades.

With this in mind, here are a few nutrients that count. Some will help your circulation, some will help your brain, and some will help in the stimulation of your pituitary function.

These substances fall into several categories:

❑ Herbal substances
❑ Food concentrates
❑ Vitamins
❑ Minerals
❑ Prescription medicine with alternative use

Let's take a look.

Herbal Substances

Ginkgo Biloba. The leaves of our planet's oldest living tree provide an extract whose remarkable effects have made it one of the most widely used and thoroughly researched herbal substances. In December 1992, *Lancet*, the premier British medical journal, reported that nineteen out of forty European medical studies had found significant to major improvements in the mental function of older patients put on ginkgo biloba extract for anywhere from six weeks to three months. Ginkgo almost certainly improves circulation to the brain.

Studies as far back as the 1970s show a consistent increase in capillary and venous blood flow to the head in elderly patients. Indeed, in some studies, the response seems to be greatest in precisely those patients suffering the most severe symptoms of cerebral circulatory insufficiency. I don't believe, however, that this indicates ginkgo won't be beneficial to most of us who merely have reached middle age. For one thing, ginkgo has powerful protective functions as an antioxidant. It's a voracious scavenger of deadly free radicals, and its marked affinity for the central nervous system promises brain protection—and that is not only highly desirable but hard to come by since the blood brain barrier deters many useful antioxidants from reaching the brain.

Circulation is also critical to the function of the heart and the sexual organs. Nothing moves efficiently without a good blood supply. In the case of sex function, the effects of ginkgo are increasingly well documented. Whether the primary mechanism is due to a direct local vasodilating effect on circulation in the penis or whether improvements are caused by a change in central nervous system reflexes or even a change in pituitary function is not known. It is quite possible that there is an integration of all three mechanisms.

On the pituitary side there is good evidence that ginkgo stimulates dopamine synthesis, and dopamine (see below) is itself a powerful stimulator of pituitary function.

If you take ginkgo, be sure to take a formulation that contains a 24-percent concentration of extract. Weaker extracts are not effective. A standard dosage is 40 to 60 mg daily. Regular users of aspirin or NSAIDS, like ibuprofen, should be cautious about combining them with ginkgo, since all of these substances inhibit platelet activity, i.e., reduce clotting—and, if there is any bleeding going on, could dangerously increase it.

Ginseng. Ginseng is a remarkable herb extracted from a plant grown in North America, South America, and many parts of Asia. Over the years, ginseng has gained a solid reputation for stimulating the aging body. Improved sexuality, energy, alertness, and resistance to stress have been reported. Highly prized for these benefits, it was expensive because of its rarity. Now, however, because of the discovery of worldwide sources, it is found in most pharmacies and health food stores. It has been shown to be a direct pituitary stimulant and, according to the evidence of a number of well-conducted studies, has positive effects on mental functioning. Though specific effects on testosterone production are not known, it most likely has some stimulating effect on production in view of the improvements reported in sexuality. Ginseng comes in various forms: capsules of powder, liquid extracts, and concentrates. Though dosage is not well documented, standard preparations should be obtained from reliable companies.

L-Dopa. L-Dopa is an amino acid found in protein foods that the body uses to make dopamine. Dopamine, in turn, is one of the more important neurotransmitters; it makes possible the transfer of information from neuron to neuron in the brain.

Some researchers believe a decline may be in part responsible for the faltering ability of the hypothalamic/pituitary axis to stimulate testosterone production as men age. Dopamine deficiency has been shown to cause a decline in hypothalamic releasing factors.

L-Dopa is most widely used for the treatment of a dreadful dopamine deficiency disease called Parkinson's. In this disease, the *substantia nigra*, an area in the lower part of the brain, degenerates resulting in decreased local production of dopamine. Treatment with L-Dopa can reverse the declining levels for some years.

Interestingly, deficiency in testosterone in men has been frequently documented in Parkinson's disease, though it is rarely added to treatment of the condition outside of my practice. One of the earliest reported "side effects" of L-Dopa was the observed increase in sexually oriented behaviors. Nurses soon learned to guard their fannies and were on the alert for more overt displays of sexuality. L-Dopa has also been used successfully to treat anorgasmia, a lack of ability to have a normal orgasm, particularly in women. I have seen this work in my patients.

With your doctor's assistance, you may wish to consider L-dopa supplementation as you climb into late middle-age. It is a prescription medicine (even though it is a natural nutritional supplement) that may not be compatible with certain medicines. A nightly tablet of 100 mg (taken with juice alone) is a typical dose. Those who are interested in a do-it-yourself approach might consider that fish is high in L-dopa and up their dietary intake.

Vitamins

Vitamin C. Readers will be glad to learn that this most famous of the vitamins enhances the pituitary gland's responsiveness to changes in hormone levels. In cases where midlife changes in testosterone levels are caused by pituitary sluggishness, this increased activity can raise testosterone levels. And, with the efficiency that the body so often shows when everything is humming along nicely, high testosterone levels have themselves been found to raise vitamin C levels by a mechanism of action which is not yet understood. Good health reinforces itself.

Conversely, low levels of vitamin C have been found to increase levels of aromatase, the principle agent for converting testosterone to estrogen. Clearly, you should keep your vitamin C levels up.

It has also been known for many years that vitamin C is essential for the formation of the basic steroid hormones of the adrenal glands and of the gonads in both sexes. What is equally fascinating to me is the connection of vitamin C to the circulatory system. I don't mean merely its familar antioxidant protection capacities. Two-time Nobel Prize winner Linus Pauling suggested that vitamin C and L-lysine are involved in collagen synthesis and are essential to maintaining normal blood vessels and connective tissue. He presented dramatic case histories of the reversal of serious circulatory symptoms with the use of high doses of both substances.

There is probably no need for me to mention all of the other beneficial effects stimulated by this peerless vitamin. The days when many doctors dissuaded their patients from taking vitamin C supplements are long past. More and more medical professionals have read Enstrom's study showing that the difference between population groups that merely eat a healthy diet and population groups that eat a healthy diet and also supplement with vitamin C is that the latter group—the vitamin takers—have far lower rates of cancer and heart disease. This was no small study. Enstrom was using the fruits of a database that had followed the health and mortality of 11,348 adults for more than a decade.

I generally encourage my patients to take approximately one to three grams of vitamin C a day. Although this is a "mega-dose," there are no studies indicating adverse effects at this level, and animals that produce their own vitamin C manufacture at least the body weight equivalent of that dose.

Vitamin E. Vitamin E was first shown to enhance potency in rodents who had been made deficient. Human studies have been less supportive as a direct treatment. However, E's effect as an antioxidant capable of reducing cardiovascular disease and offering neuro-protection from adverse changes in the aging brain certainly point toward an anti-aging role and possibly some inhibition of hormonal decline. The recent World Symposium on vitamin E came to the unequivocal conclusion that the amounts found in the human diet are not enough to provide the full range of vitamin E's antioxidant effects. I believe 400 to 800 I.U.s a day is sufficient for most adults.

B Complex Vitamins. All of the B vitamins are important in cellular functions. The B vitamin most likely to be beneficial for pituitary functions is Pyridoxine (Vitamin B_6) because of its ability to decrease the secretion of prolactin, an inhibitor of the gonadotrophins.

Folic acid and B_{12} are also important Bs because they, like Pyridoxine, facilitate the clearance of homocysteine, a critical substance produced as part of the recycling of the body's amino acids. Experts now think that a buildup of homocysteine in the bloodstream leads to blockage in our arteries. It has been estimated that one-third of all strokes and heart attacks are the result of excess homocysteine in the blood. But the significant fact is that almost all cases of elevated homocysteine can be lowered into the normal range simply by supplementing with the simple, cheap, and nontoxic B vitamins. A few people with a genetic predisposition to high homocysteine levels require much higher doses or the addition of other nutrients. If you have the tests recommended in the last chapter, your doctor will be able to determine whether you need higher nutritional doses.

Minerals

Zinc. Of all the minerals, zinc still stands out because of the classic deficiency studies that demonstrated the dramatic interference with normal hypothalamic/pituitary function caused by its lack. Severe deficiency literally halted the changes of puberty in teenage boys, effects which rapidly reversed when zinc was restored to normal levels. There would be little need to write about such bizarre situations if zinc deficiency were rare. But National Health and Nutrition Surveys—NHANES I, II, and III—performed over the last thirty years have consistently shown deficient intake in large segments of our society, particularly the aging population.

Aggravating deficits of zinc are the effects of alcohol and medication; in particular, the thiazide diuretics primarily used for treating hypertension and fluid retention. There are studies linking lower testosterone and increased problems of impotence with their use.

Zinc's other major role, which we discussed in detail in Chapter 5, is its inhibitory effects on aromatase enzyme activity. (See "Changing the Testosterone/Estrogen Balance" on page 190.)

Food Concentrates

Resveratrol. Resveratrol is a recently discovered grape skin extract, made from certain varieties of red grapes, which has been reported to be one of the key substances that gives grapes and wine protective health benefits—including cancer protection and reduction of cardiovascular disease and strokes. Equally exciting is the fact that resveratrol improves the functioning of the liver P450 system, allowing the body to more effectively remove excess estrogen. Resveratrol and grape seed extract are also excellent antioxidants, measured to be fifty times more potent than vitamin E!

Soy Extracts. See "Changing the Testosterone/Estrogen Balance" on page 190 for a discussion of these important nutritional substances.

Prescription Medicine With Alternative Use

Seligiline. In addition to L-dopa, there is another drug, Seligiline, (often sold under the name Eldepryl), that is also commonly used in the treatment of Parkinson's disease and which, like L-dopa, appears to boost levels of testosterone by exerting an influence on the control panel in the brain. Although Seligiline has many highly positive and widely documented effects on human health, its effect on testosterone levels is my own discovery, and I have watched it work in dozens of patients. Testosterone levels sometimes go from subnormal or borderline levels to the upper normal ranges. The clinical effects of testosterone increase—increased energy, strength, stamina, mental sharpness, and sexual interest and responsiveness—are also consistently observed.

Some other notable effects of Seligiline include the following:

❏ It increases the production of dopamine, hence its use in treating Parkinson's disease.
❏ It stimulates the cells in the brain to increase brain repair processes, a vital aspect of anti-aging treatments. Part of the problem with secondary hypogonadism is very likely to involve subtle damage to the control panel cells in the hypothalamus.
❏ Presumably as a result of the effects just described, Seligiline has a well-observed effect of increasing cognitive function and overall mental sharpness. It also has mild antidepressant effects.
❏ Animal studies show increased sexuality as well as an association in the animals studied between that and increased longevity.
❏ It shows powerful, protective antioxidant effects; in particular, the ability to control the oxidation of LDL cholesterol.

A Multitude of Approaches

I hope you will do most of the good things I've just discussed and observe your body carefully after you've done them. You will probably see significant improvements in your energy level and possibly other improvements as well. But you still may not experience everything you've come to this book hoping to recover. You may not get that jolt of youthfulness, of dynamic physical force, of sexual vigor that you were really looking for. I don't know your age, of course, and can't predict your physical condition, but I do expect that many of my readers will already be experiencing the midlife blahs. The gray zone of the male menopause will have sunk a hook or two into your vulnerable aging body. In other words, your hormone levels are falling and your quality of life is going down with them.

In that case, what you're going to have to do is move on to the next stages of the treatment program. You're going to have to take very positive steps to improve the hormonal balance in your body. Naturally, any such treatment plan should start at the conservative end. As you know, I am thoroughly committed to the safety and desirability of testosterone replacement when needed, but it is always better to let the body do its own work, if possible.

So—since there are many more ways to skin the hormonal cat than one—here is the triad of hormonal approaches, from the least interventional to the most, that we are going to discuss:

1) Restore your hormone balance by altering the testosterone/estrogen ratio in favor of testosterone.
2) Administer chorionic gonadotrophin in order to stimulate testicular production of testosterone.
3) Replace testosterone directly by any one of a number of modes.

Let's consider these choices one by one.

Changing the Testosterone/Estrogen Balance

As I explained in Chapter 5, one of the most significant contributors to the male menopause is a changing ratio of testosterone to estrogen as men age. The concept upon which this book is founded—*windows of optimum hormonal function and balance*—is violated when that ratio alters, and the man who thought at forty that he would be young forever finds out at fifty that he isn't the man he was.

A relative excess of estrogen to testosterone dampens down male sexuality, increases risk factors for heart disease, blocks the effective action of testosterone in all the areas of the body, and inhibits the hypothalamic/pituitary axis.

If, upon testing your hormone levels, you discover a relatively high estrogen level—for most men that will be anything above 30 ng/dl—here is a quick review of the steps you should take (hopefully after giving your doctor a xerox copy of Chapter 5 and pleading/insisting that he read it).

❏ Take supplemental zinc—approximately 50 mg twice daily until you see improvement, and then 50 mg daily. Zinc inhibits levels of aromatase, the testosterone-to-estrogen conversion enzyme. Many men will restore a proper balance of testosterone to estrogen purely through the use of zinc.

❏ If you're significantly overweight, find a good diet and tighten your belt. In both men and women, fat cells are full of aromatase and tend to store plentiful quantities of estrogen. As the pounds fall off, so will your estrogen conversion activity and many of the symptoms of the male menopause will vanish as well.

❏ If you've fallen into a pattern of fairly heavy drinking—I don't mean you have to be an alcoholic—you are aggravating your natural midlife problem of staying in the window of optimal hormonal function. Alcohol significantly inhibits the clearance of estrogen from the bloodstream and also decreases zinc levels. I encourage my patients not to have more than one or two drinks a day. Unfortunately, in cases where the estrogen component of a man's hormonal problem seems dominant, I may have to ask a patient to give up drinking altogether. As you can imagine, for some men this becomes a sticking point.

❑ A high consumption of soy protein has been associated with many healthful effects, including lower rates of certain kinds of cancer. For our purposes, the chief importance of soy is that it is high in isoflavones, a type of phytoestrogen very similar in chemical structure to human estrogens but far weaker. Typically such estrogens have only about 1/500 the active effect of estradiol, the most active human estrogen. High levels of phytoestrogens compete with the female hormone for receptor sites in your body, block its actions—which can include some inhibition of pituitary functions—and stimulate the P450 system in the liver to more actively process and excrete excess estrogen.

Two other food supplements have positive and negative significance. Grapefruit—wonderful fruit that it is—may be an enemy of men in the gray zone for it tends to inhibit the liver's breakdown of estrogen. Cruciferous vegetables, such as broccoli and cauliflower, on the other hand, stimulate the burning-off of extra estrogen.

Capsules of both isoflavones and cruciferous vegetables are available now and may help those of you who are always on the run to increase your intake. Doses are individually determined, since these are foods. But they really help!

❑ Check out the list of prescription drugs in Appendix 3 that increase estrogen or inhibit testosterone. If you're on any of them, see if your doctor can devise a substitute that isn't on the list.

Ten to twenty percent of my male menopausal patients experience virtually a full recovery by taking these steps alone. This is usually an indication that their testosterone level was adequate, and the problem is estrogen. Once the estrogen is under control, we will sometimes notice a beneficial rise in the free testosterone level. Certainly, for all my hormonal patients, the steps previously outlined are recommended. And yet, as one can see from the percentages just quoted, in the majority of men the improvements experienced are not sufficient. It's necessary to raise their testosterone levels also. Let's look at the least interventional method of doing just that.

Chorionic Gonadotrophin

Chorionic gonadotrophin is very similar in molecular structure and function to LH, one of the main stimulating hormones produced by the pituitary gland. You may recall our discussion of gonadotrophins in Chapter 4. These are the substances—appropriately enough—that send messages to the gonads. When your pituitary, for instance, receives word from the hypothalamus that testosterone levels are too low, it secretes a gonadotrophin such as LH or FSH which, arriving at the testicles, transmits a message to the Leydig cells down there that roughly translates as, "Come on, guys, coffee break is over. Time to get back on the job." At least, that's the way things are supposed to work.

However, if a man's testosterone levels are too low, clearly something is broken. An experienced endocrinologist quickly asks himself a basic question: is the deficiency that this man shows due to lack of stimulation from the control centers in the brain, or does it result from testicular incapacity to secrete sufficient male hormone? In medical terms, he wants to know if the deficiency is caused by secondary or primary hypogonadism.

Usually, if it's a control center problem, lab tests will show that levels of LH and FSH are low, indicating that the body is not making an effort to stimulate testosterone increase. If it's a problem of testicular incapacity, LH and FSH levels will be high because the pituitary, in a vain effort to force the testicles to manufacture testosterone adequately, will be releasing those hormones at every opportunity.

Although the distinction sounds simple, measuring and interpreting these hormone levels can be complex. I have usually found that one can test the situation through treatment.

A hormone called chorionic gonadotrophin is an injectable booster that sends the same message to the gonads as LH or FSH and, since it's more easily manufactured, we use it to stimulate testicular production. Frequently, the best approach is to simply give chorionic gonadotrophin to the testosterone-deficient male and see what happens. You will generally see a rise in testosterone within a month after first administration of chorionic gonadotrophin, if the testosterone problem was due to insufficient stimulation from the control centers. The Leydig cells within the testicles will increase in size and very often the testicles themselves will actually grow larger.

Used for years to boost fertility in males and to help in cases of undescended testicles, chorionic gonadotrophin has long been overlooked as a specific treatment for testosterone deficiency. In my own progress treating patients in the male menopause, CG has been the newest and one of the brightest threads. The simplicity, naturalness, and safety has been so great that the use of this treatment has totally changed my approach.

Chorionic gonadotrophin is administered by injection. The syringes and needles are equivalent to those used for insulin injections—they are extremely small, 30-gauge (about the diameter of a human hair!), only one inch long, and virtually painless. The rankest amateur around can give them with a minimum of training. The injections are usually given two to three times weekly.

Your physician can easily work out an individualized dose to bring testosterone response back into the normal, healthy range. CG works nicely with other natural boosters and, in early stages of the male menopause, is often only needed to give an initial cycling boost to the endocrine system. The pituitary continues on after this shove in the normal direction activates control panel receptors.

A high percentage of patients, especially in their midlife years, have a satisfactory response to chorionic gonadotrophin. Testosterone levels will frequently rise into the 600 to 800 ng/dl range.

As men get older, the effectiveness of chorionic gonadotrophin may decline. In other words, the older a man is the more likely it is that he has developed actual testicular incapacity, i.e., an incapacity of the Leydig cells to produce sufficient quantities of male hormone no matter how sharply they're stimulated by pituitary gonadotrophins. It is rare to see a man in his forties or fifties with testicular incapacity. But once that stage is reached—whether young or old—it's time to move on to the next stage: actual hormone replacement.

Testosterone Replacement—A Medley of Modes

There are five principal methods of testosterone replacement: injections, lozenges, patches, gels and creams, and pellets. As I've said before, injections are the least effective form of testosterone replacement, and I no longer recommend them. But let's look at these delivery systems one by one.

Injections. This is still the most common method of replacing testosterone, and it is infinitely the worst. Most negative medical studies on testosterone use were conducted using injections. Unfortunately, this mode of replacement raises testosterone levels far to abruptly and often to a nonphysiologic height. This not only very poorly imitates the body's own pattern, but frequently causes a rebound effect in the form of increased estrogen levels. Since there are no advantages to the use of injections, this entire mode of replacement is ripe for the trash can.

Lozenges. This is an excellent method of increasing testosterone. The chief drawback is that five or six hours after a lozenge is swallowed, hormone levels begin to fall again. Therefore, one must usually take the lozenge three times a day, and some men are annoyed at having to build this into their schedule. If that is not a problem, this is the simplest and most convenient method of male hormone replacement. Hormone levels can usually be brought up to the 500 to 1,000 ng/dl range. The method of administration also partially mimics the natural pulsatile release of hormone. Testosterone lozenges are not yet sold to the general public; what you'll need to do is have your physician prescribe them for you and have them made by a compounding pharmacy. Compounding pharmacies—of which, fortunately, there are an ever-growing number—can put together medications in whatever form a medical doctor considers desirable.

Patches. Testosterone patches were a highly useful development in the war on the male menopause. They can be placed just about anywhere on the body; they provide a slow, steady release of hormone; and they are essentially side-effect free. At least, if your skin can take it. Some men get rashes from the adhesive material that keeps the patch sticking to the skin. And, since the patch must be changed daily and it usually leaves a red circle on the skin that lasts for a while, some men are resentful of the polka dot effect. I have also found that patches can usually only get men up into the 500 to 600 ng/dl range. This is fine for some men. Others, who were presumably high testosterone males in their youth, find that this brings only a very partial relief from symptoms. Nonetheless, the patch is an excellent delivery system for men who only need a moderate boost in their testosterone level and who are undetered by its cosmetic disadvantages.

Gels and Creams. These are also convenient and highly effective methods of administering testosterone. Both gels and creams are rapidly absorbed through any skin surface. Repeated use on one skin area will increase hairiness there, so it's best to rotate one's spots. Both gels and creams are convenient to use. The gels disappear into the skin quickly and the creams do also, much like a moisturizing cream or a hand cream. They should be used once or twice daily, depending upon the dosage you and your physician desire. I usually recommend twice daily—morning and night. Both preparations should have a strength of 25 mg per gram of base. On a twice-daily schedule, rub in one half-gram in the morning and one half-gram at night. Men who are using this form of testosterone to improve sexual function may wish to use the cream (not the gel—it will sting) on the head or shaft of the penis or on the scrotum. This delivers testosterone in a more concentrated form into the genital area. In addition, because there are tremendous concentrations of the 5-alpha reductase enzyme down there, much of this testosterone will be converted to dihydro-testosterone (DHT), a form of the enzyme that cannot be converted by aromatase into estrogen. Some doctors believe DHT provokes prostate trouble, but DHT creams are prescribed and sold widely in Europe, and European studies have shown no increase in prostate problems as a result of their use. The only disadvantage I have noticed in the use of testosterone creams and gels is that *discipline* and *accuracy* are required in measuring the amount to apply each day. If those words are not in your personality profile, or if you have an ingrained tendency to think that more is always better, then you're probably better off using some other method of hormone replacement.

Pellets. Discovering pellets was a significant stage for me as I treated testosterone-deficient patients. It more or less coincided with my realization that injections were a truly ineffective modality of treatment, and it offered another method of offering long-term treatment with a minimum of patient inconvenience. Injections have usually been given once every three or four weeks. Pellets need to be implanted only once every four to six months. These little gel-like objects are inserted into the buttocks—a minor and completely painless procedure (a painkiller is used). Imbedded in the fat, the testosterone formulation gradually dissolves, giving a slow, steady constant infusion of the hormone into the body. The vast majority of men treated with pellets find this delivery system extremely effective—usually more effective than anything else they've tried. It is usually not difficult to get a man into the 600 to 900 ng/dl range and keep him there. Moreover, estrogen conversion does not occur at high rates. For some reason, the human body creates far more estrogen from testosterone when the testosterone is delivered in a large surge than when it gradually enters the system.

If you and your physician decide to try pellets, he should contact Bartor Phamacal in Rye, New York. To my knowledge, this company is the only FDA-approved maker of testosterone pellets in the United States. The cost, when calculated by the year, is somewhat less than patches or lozenges.

A Hormone Progression

I believe we are going to find, as male hormone therapy becomes increasingly widespread, that many men will actually progress over two or three decades through all the stages of hormonal manipulation. In their forties or fifties, they may be correcting for a rise in estrogen relative to testosterone. Some years later, their doctor may suggest they take chorionic gonadotrophin to stimulate their own production of the male hormone. And, in the final stage of hormone therapy, they will actually move on to testosterone replacement in the form that is most convenient and effective for them.

Changing body, changing treatment. There is a certain elegance and simplicity about this approach. You will get older, your hormone levels will decline, and you will show symptoms. But this will no longer be mysterious to you. I think you know what to do.

CHAPTER 14:
Conclusion

What are people capable of as they grow older? A patient of mine, Henry Williams, represents a sort of answer. I'm sure Henry was always quite a physical specimen. When he was young, he was a professional golfer competing on the PGA tour. Now that he's eighty, he naturally only competes in senior events. I—who all my life have been a passionate golfer—sometimes play a round with Henry. If I'm playing my best, I might beat him. But usually it's wallet-whipping time for me. Henry is my hero.

Henry went down to Florida two years ago to compete in the PGA Half Century Tournament—that's for golfers who have been members of the Professional Golf Association for fifty years or more. He won the tournament . . . by seven strokes.

In other words, my sometime golf partner is the Tiger Woods of the senior set.

Since Henry is my patient, I was naturally very curious about the hormone levels of a man who's so phenomenally vigorous and athletic at an age when most of us are content to simply set the rocker in motion and flick on the remote control. I first measured Henry's testosterone three years ago. It was 749 ng/dl. That set me thinking. I don't think I'd ever measured a testosterone level in a man Henry's age that was quite that high.

Last spring, when he returned from Florida, Henry remarked that he hadn't been feeling himself lately. He fatigued more easily, he had lost eight or nine pounds off of his already sinewy frame, and, worst thing of all, he often felt plumb tuckered-out at the end of eighteen holes. By Henry's remarkable standards, he was feeling pretty rotten.

He came in for some tests, and one thing stood out: Henry's testosterone was now 423 ng/dl. Perfectly normal for a man his age—but I knew it wasn't normal for Henry. A few weeks later, after a thorough workup to rule out prostate cancer and other problems, I implanted some testosterone pellets in Henry and stood back to see what would happen. A little cough and a sputter, and the old engine roared into action. As Henry put it recently, "I feel like eighty going on sixty. When I finish eighteen holes of golf, I'm not tired . . . I'm pretty sure I could do another eighteen."

Talk to Henry at the end of an active day, and you're in the presence of a man full of self-confidence, energy, and wit, not to mention uncommon mental and physical vitality—exactly where we would all like to be at his age.

I know you understand what happened to Henry for that brief period last year: he hit the male menopause—or it hit him. It came a little late. Most men run into their hormonal nemesis when they're in their forties, fifties, or sixties.

The point is what it always is for men: hormonal individuality. Your hormones will decline according to a schedule that only they know. My advice to you is don't submit. Take action! There's no reason why you should allow yourself to become a caricature of the person you once were.

If you approach the challenges of age with that attitude and this book in your hand, I firmly believe you will have an excellent chance of sailing through the second half of life. Or, as Henry Williams said to me the other day, "If the next fifty years are as good as the last fifty years, I'll be all right!"

Appendix 1:

Nonhormonal Approaches to Sexual Dysfunction

No Stone Unturned

Here, together with a brief review of the hormonal approach to erectile dysfunction, are some other approaches that are complementary to it. Sexuality—like almost everything else in the human body—works best when just about everything is working perfectly. We can't really have that as we get older, so we have to settle for the next best thing: having almost everything working nearly as well as it can. That's why it doesn't make sense, in the long term, to deal with aging by adding one pill, or one hormone, or one lifestyle change. The best results ensue when one adds quite a lot of improvements.

So let's assume you're a man who would like his sexual equipment to go on functioning for nine or ten decades. Here are some of the approaches you and your doctor should consider.

1) If testing shows that your testosterone levels are less than ideal—which is very different from deficient—consider testosterone replacement using physiologic doses of testosterone in the patch, pill, or pellet form, so that they do not overconvert to E2/E1 estrogens. See Chapter 13 for guidelines.

2) If your estrogen levels are at all elevated (over 30 ng/dl) use the natural aromatase inhibitors such as zinc as described in Chapter 5.

3) Once again, turn to Chapter 5 for guidance in how to restore the P450 liver system so that it can effectively clear estrogen and hormonal byproducts such as epitestosterone, which has been suspected to be a testosterone blocker.

4) Rehabilitate the levator ani muscles with regular Kegel exercises—see Appendix 2.

5) Review any medications you may be on with your personal physician and compare them with the list in Appendix 3.

6) Ask your doctor to help you test out the effectiveness of various substances, which by different methods augment the functioning of the penis:

   ❑ Try some of nature's natural vasodilators. For instance, ginkgo biloba extract made from the leaves of the ginkgo tree. One 1992 article in the premier British medical journal *Lancet* reported that thirty-nine out of forty European medical studies found significant to major improvements in the mental function of older patients after they took ginkgo extract for six weeks to three months. Ginkgo improves circulation to the brain and apparently also to the legs and many other parts of the body. When Dr. Sikora and his colleagues gave ginkgo to sixty impotent men, they noticed improvements in the majority of them after six to eight weeks. After six months, potency had been regained by 50 percent of the men. (Sikora, R. et al., "Ginkgo biloba extract in the therapy of erectile dysfunction," *Journal of Urology*, 1989;141:188A.)

   Garlic is also important because it helps to unblock the arteries. In India, in the mid-1980s, Dr. Gupta Sainani and his researchers at the Poona Medical College discovered that platelet clumping and fibrin activity decreased in direct proportion to garlic consumption.

❑ Your doctor may wish to try yohimbine, a drug made from the West African yohimbe tree. The only drug approved by the FDA for potency problems, yohimbine is thought to block adrenergic neurotransmitters thereby stopping the sympathetic nerves from inhibiting the erection. Yohimbine also promotes the flow of arterial blood to the penis. The drug has numerous side effects, including dizziness, headaches, and elevations in blood pressure and heart rate and should be taken under careful medical supervision.

❑ Damiana leaf is an herb frequently found in Chinese herbal remedies. It has been reputed to enhance sexual activity although, to my knowledge, extensive research has not been done on it. The best blends appear to combine saw palmetto with Damiana.

❑ Muira-puama is a native folk medicine of Brazil that for several centuries has had a reputation as an aphrodisiac. It appears to have genuine effects. European researchers reported in 1990 on 262 patients with inability to attain or maintain an erection. Within two weeks of receiving a daily dose of Muira-puama extract (1 to 1.5 grams), 62 percent reported significant recovery of function. The mechanism of action is unknown. Muira-puama can be obtained in health food stores and does not appear to have side effects when taken in conservative doses.

This is actually only a small sampling of the current approaches to impotence. Urologists will have numerous further suggestions, including penile implants and various mechanical devices. I suggest you try some of the less invasive approaches mentioned previously first. Above all, if your testosterone levels are less than ideal, work with your doctor on your hormone levels. Bring testosterone up, keep estrogen down. Give yourself six months, and maintain a positive attitude. In too many studies, time has been the missing ingredient.

Appendix 2:

Kegel Exercises

The group of muscles that form the pelvic sling or hammock, the *levator ani*, give rise to the circular muscles that control urine, bowel, and, in females, vaginal tone. They also give rise in the male to the key muscles at the base of the penis that are critical to the tone in the pressure chambers, the *corpora cavernosa*. This complex group of muscles is highly dependent on testosterone for maintaining both substance and activity, thinning and weakening when deficiency appears. What is clear from both research and experience is that function and tone can be restored when hormonal correction and stimulation through specific exercises are followed. What I have found is that exercise without hormonal support is much less successful.

Kegel exercises, which date back to the 1950s, were specifically developed to tonify the pelvic muscles to help control urine leakage in women. Various biofeedback devices were developed to teach the individual to squeeze and strengthen the proper individual groups. More recently, research has shown that males can gain significant improvement in erectile function as well. The use of external biofeedback, however, in most cases is not necessary for success.

Envision the *levator ani* group of muscles as a web that is intimately inter-connected. Contraction of one part invariably results in tension in other parts. The hammock stretches from the pubic bone in the front to the tailbone, the coccyx, in the back. When sustained contractions occur, there is a lifting sensation in the anus and perenium, hence the name, *levator* or lifter. As contractions occur, there is muscle fiber recruitment of the other associated muscles of the anal and urethral sphincters, as well as the muscles at the base of the penis, the *bulbo-* and *ischio-cavernosa* muscles. This process can be utilized to restore control of urine leakage, tone in the vagina to improve sexual response, and increased pressure in the chambers to restore fullness to erections.

There are several types of exercises, but all require repetition and habitual maintenance for continued success.

Classically, the contraction of the muscle that stops the flow of urine will initiate contraction of the sling. By additionally squeezing the anus at the same time and holding this feeling of tension, there is a steady increase in tension throughout the sling and a lifting sensation in the perineum.

Short, intense contractions may help a portion of the muscle or the sphincters themselves, but it takes longer sustained contractions to recruit the full web of fibers that extend out to the *bulbo-* and *ischio-cavernosa* muscles.

I usually recommend that contractions lasting 10 to 15 seconds are required 15 to 20 times per day. Some researchers recommend 60 to 100 separate squeezes, a task that is hard to maintain.

I recommend that exercises be triggered by common events when distraction is not likely to interfere. Red lights while driving, commercials when viewing television or listening to the radio, and time when seated on the toilet are good repeatable situations.

For males, "bonking" squeezes when an erection is noted in the morning are an effective muscle-stimulating alternative. "Bonking" squeezes are a series of short burst-type contractions that result in bouncing or flexing the penis to lift or jump upward. This, togethter with the longer tonifying exercises, has been very effective in some cases. Also, since the *bulbo-cavernosa* muscle is involved with the sensations of contractions, which occur at the time of climax and ejaculation, there is a significant increase in pleasurable sensations at this time as a bonus.

The use of topical testosterone to the vagina and the penis will greatly increase the rebuilding of the critical muscles in these areas.

For women, a vaginal cream made up by a compounding pharmacy with Estradiol 0.25 mg/gram or Estriol 1 mg/gram plus testosterone 0.25 mg/gram in a cream base used three times weekly until response, then one to two times weekly for maintenance, 1 to 2 grams per dose, will help greatly. This same mild concentration can safely be used on any external parts to help improve sensory response as well. The vaginal cream is inserted deeply into the vagina with an applicator supplied by the pharmacy.

For men, systemic correction of testosterone levels by appropriate methods is important. Additionally, a topical testosterone cream applied to the penis and to the scrotum will sometimes result in rapid improvement in erectile function in conjunction with the exercises. This cream can also be compounded without difficulty. It should be made up with testosterone 5 mg/gram in a cream base and applied three times weekly in one-quarter-teaspoon (1 gram) doses. Application to the scrotum results in conversion of the testosterone to dihydro-testosterone (DHT), a form of hormone needed to activate receptors in the pelvic nerves, muscles, and blood vessels.

Neither of these creams should be used as a lubricant for intercourse, although in women, increased response and normalization of vaginal tissues will itself result in better natural lubrication.

Appendix 3:

Drug/Hormone Interactions

Some substances help and some interfere with proper hormone balance, level or effect. Knowing which ones have positive or negative effects can make or break an individual who has entered the gray zone of marginal hormone function. Various common substances, including medicines, foods, and nutrients can have effects on liver metabolism, which controls hormone breakdown. Since testosterone can be rapidly metabolized peripherally and by the phase I enzymes in the liver, it has a very short half-life and is therefore not as easily affected by factors which alter liver metabolism. Estrogen, however, is slowly broken down by both the phase I and phase II enzymes. Therefore, any change there will result in increased building up in the bloodstream and backing up in critical tissues.

Drugs that inhibit the P450 phase I System,
resulting in increased estrogen levels:
Pain/anti-inflammatory drugs: NSAIDS (ibuprofin, ketoprofen, and diclofenac), acetaminophen, aspirin
Propoxeyphene
Antibiotics: sulfas, tetracyclines, penicillins, cefazolins, erythromycins, floxins, isoniazid
Antifungal drugs (inhibit P450 Systems and act as testosterone receptor inhibitors): Miconazole, Itraconazole, Fluconazole, Ketoconazole
Cholesterol lowering drugs (Statins): Lovastatin, Simvistatin

Antidepressants: Fluoxitine, Fluvoxamine, Paroxetine, Sertraline

Antipsychotic medicines: Thorazine, Haloperidol

Heart and blood pressure medicine: Propranolol, Quinidine, Amiodarone (also decreases testosterone production), Coumadin, Methyldopa

Calcium channel blockers: antiacids, Omeprazole, Cimetidine

Vitamins and nutrients: high-dose vitamin E, general dietary deficiencies and malnutrition, grapefruit

Abusive substances: alcohol, amphetamines, marijuana, cocaine

Drugs or substances that may speed up
the P450 System, decreasing estrogen levels:

Vitamins: high-dose vitamin C (also increases testosterone production), vitamin K, niacin

Drugs: phenobarbital, chlordiazepoxide, carbamepazine, trazodone, sulcrafate

Foods: soy products, vegetarian diets, cruciferous vegetables (broccoli, cauliflower), shellfish (oysters), resveratrol (grape skin compound)

Some drugs and substances compete for testosterone
cellular receptors or change metabolism indirectly:

Antifungal drugs: (as above)

Pesticides, Spironolacone, some cancer chemotherapy drugs, Thiazide diuretics, DHEA

Notes

Chapter 2

1. Heller, C. G. and Myers, G. B., "The male climacteric, its symptomatology, diagnosis and treatment," *Journal of the American Medical Association*, 1944; 126(8): 472-477.

For more recent considerations of the effects of androgen decline in aging males see:
Harman, S. M. and Blackman, M. R., "Male menopause, myth or menace," *The Endocrinologist*, 1994; 4(3): 212-217. *Also:* Swerdloff, R. S. and Wang, C., "Androgen deficiency and aging in men," *Western Journal of Medicine*, 1993; 159(5): 579-585. *Also:* Vermuelen, A. "Androgens in the aging male," *Journal of Clinical Endocrinology and Metabolism*, 1991; 73(2): 221-224. *Also:* Mooradian, A. D. et al., "Biological actions of androgens," *Endocrine Reviews*, 1987; 8(1): 1-28.

For general discussion of the effects of testosterone replacement see:
Tenover, J., "Androgen administration to aging men," *Clinical Andrology*, 1994; 23(4): 877-892. *Also:* Tenover, J. S., "Effects of testosterone supplementation in the aging male," *Journal of Clinical Endocriniology and Metabolism*, 1992; 74(4): 1092-1098. *Also:* Weksler, M. E., "Hormone replacement for men: has the time come?" *Geriatrics*, 1995; 50(10): 52-55. *Also:* Bardin, C. W. et al., "Androgens: risks and benefits," *Journal of Clinical Endocriniology and Metabolism*, 1991; 73(1): 4-7. *Also:* Bhasin, S. and Bremner, W. J., "Emerging issues in androgen replacement therapy," *Journal of Clinical Endocrinology and Metabolism*, 1997; 82(1): 3-8.

Chapter 4

1. *AACE Clinical Practice Guidelines for the Evaluation and Treatment of Hypogonadism in Adult Male Patients*, American Association of Clinical Endocrinologists, 1993

Chapter 6

1. Tobin, C. and Pecot-Dechavassine, M., "Effect of castration on the morphology of the motor end-plates of the rat levator ani muscle," *European Journal of Cellular Biology*, 1982; 26(2): 284-288. *See also:* Vyskocil, F. and Gutmann, E., "Electrophysiological and contractile properties of the levator ani muscle after castration and testosterone administration," Pflugers Archives, 1977; 368(1-2): 105-109. *Also:* Souccar, C., et al., "The influence of testosterone on neuromuscular transmission in hormone sensitive mammalian skeletal muscles," *Muscle Nerve*, 1982; 5(3): 232-237. *Also:* Sachs, B. D., "Role of striated penile muscles in penile reflexes, copulation, and induction of pregnancy in the rat," *Journal of Reproductive Fertility*, 1982; 66(2): 433-443.

2. Kaiser, F. et al., "Impotence and aging: clinical and hormonal factors," *Journal of the American Geriatric Society*, 1988; 36: 511-519.

3. Claes, H. and Baert, I., "Pelvic floor exercises versus surgery in the treatment of impotence," *British Journal of Urology*, 1993; 71(1): 52-57. *See also:* Claes, H. et al., "Pelvic-perineal rehabilitation for dysfunctioning erections. A clinical and anatomophysiologic study," *International Journal of Impotence Research*, 1993; 5(1): 13-26.

4. Chamness, S. L. et al., "The effect of androgen on nitric oxide synthase in the male reproductive tract of the rat," *Fertility and Sterility*, 1995; 63(5): 1101-1107. *See also:* Zvara, P. et al., "Nitric oxide mediated erectile activity in a testosterone dependent event: a rat erection model," *International Journal of Impotence Research*, 1995; 7(4): 209-219.

5. Rajfer, J. et al., "Nitric oxide as a mediator of relaxation of the corpus cavernosum in response to nonadrenergic, noncholinergic neurotransmission," *New England Journal of Medicine*, 1992; 326(2): 90-94.

6. Chiu, A.W. et al., "Penile brachial index in impotent patients with coronary artery disease," *European Urology*, 1991; 19(3): 213-216. *See also:* Lochmann, A. et al., "Erectile dysfunction of arterial origin as possible primary manifestation of atherosclerosis," *Minerva Cardioangiol*, 1996; 44(5): 243-246.

Chapter 7

1. Zgliczynski, S. et al., "Effect of testosterone replacement therapy on lipids and lipoproteins in hypogonadic and elderly men," *Atherosclerosis*, 1996; 121(1): 35-43.

2. Chou, T. M. et al., "Testosterone induces dilation of canine coronary conductance and resistance arteries in vivo," *Circulation*, 1996; 94(10): 2614-2619. *See also:* Costarella, C. E. et al., "Testosterone causes direct relaxation of rat thoracic aorta," *Journal of Pharmacol Exp Ther*, 1996; 277(1): 34-39. *Also:* Yue, P. et al., "Testosterone relaxes rabbit coronary arteries and aorta," *Circulation*, 1995; 91(4): 1154-1160.

3. Philips, G. B. et al., "Sex hormones and hemostatic risk factors for cornoary heart disease in men with hypertension," *Journal of Hypertension*, 1993; 11(7): 699-702. *See also:* Jeppesen, L. L. et al., "Decreased serum testosterone in men with acute ischemic stroke," *Arterioscler Thromb Vasc Biol*, 1996; 16(6): 749-754.

4. Tibblin, G. et al., "The pituitary-gonadal axis and health in elderly men: a study of men born in 1913," *Diabetes*, 1996; 45(11); 1605-1609. *See also:* "Low levels of sex hormone-binding globulin and testosterone predict the development of non-insulin-dependent diabetes in men. MRFIT Research Group. Multiple Risk Factor Intervention Trial," *American Journal of Epidemiology*, 1996; 143(9): 889-897. *Also:* Erfurth, E. M. and Hagmar, "Decreased serum testosterone and free triiodothyronine levels in healthy middle-aged men indicate an age effect at the pituitary level," *European Journal of Endocrinology*, 1995; 132(6): 663-667.

5. Marin, P. et al., "Androgen treatment of middle-aged, obese men: effects on metabolism, muscle and adipose tissues," *European Journal of Medicine*, 1992; 1(6): 329-336. *See also:* Kay-Tee Khaw et al., "Lower endogenous

androgens predict central adiposity in men," *Annals of Epidemiology*, 1992; 2(5): 675-682.

6. Philips, G. B. et al., "The association of hyperestrogenemia with coronary thrombosis in men," *Arterioscler Thromb Vasc Biol*, 1996;16(11);1383-1387.

7. Simon, D. et al., "Association between plasma total testosterone and cardiovascular risk factors in healthy adult men: the Telecom study," *Journal of Clinical Endocrinology and Metabolism*, 1997; 82(2): 682-685. *See also:* Marques-Vidal, P. et al., "Relationships of plasminogen activator inhibitor activity and lipoprotein(a) with insulin, testosterone, 17 beta-estradiol, and testosterone binding globulin in myocardial infarction patients and healthy controls," *Journal of Clinical Endocrinology and Metabolism*, 1995; 80(6): 1794-1798.

8. Glueck, C. J. et al., "Endogenous testosterone, fibrinolysis, and coronary heart disease risk in hyperlipidemic men," *Journal of Laboratory Clinical Medicine*, 1993; 122(4): 412-420.

9. Kosasih, J. B. et al., "Serum insulin-like growth factor-I and serum testosterone status of elderly men in an inpatient rehabilitation unit," *American Journal of Medical Science*, 1996; 311(4): 169-173.

10. Bjorntorp, P., "Endocrine insufficiency and nutrition in aging," *Aging* (Milano), 1993; 5(2 Suppl 1): 45-49. *See also:* Tenover, J. S., "Effects of testosterone supplementation in the aging male," *Journal of Clinical Endocrinology and Metabolism*, 1992; 75(4): 1092-1098.

11. Poggi, U. L. et al., "Plasma testosterone and serum lipids in male survivors of myocardial infarction," *Journal of Steroid Biochemistry*, 1976; 7: 229-231.

12. Lichtenstein, M. J. et al., "Sex hormones, insulin, lipids, and prevalent ischemic heart disease," *American Journal of Epidemiology*, 1987; 126(4): 647-657.

13. Philips, G. B. et al., "The association of hypotestosteronemia with coronary artery disease in men," *Arteriosclerosis and Thrombosis*, 1994; 14(5): 701-706.

14. Wu, S. and Weng, X., "Therapeutic effects of an androgenic preparation on myocardial ischemia and cardiac function in 62 elderly male coronary heart disease patients," *Chinese Medical Journal*, 1993; 106: 415.

15. Moller, J. and Einfeldt, H., *Testosterone Treatment of Cardiovascular Diseases*, Springer-Verlag, (Berlin), 1984.

16. Simon, D. et al., "Interrelation between plasma testosterone and plasma insulin in healthy adult men: the Telecom Study," *Diabetologia*, 1992; 35(2): 173-177. *See also:* Haffner, S. M. et al., "Decreased testosterone and dehydropeiandrosterone sulfate concentrations are associated with increased insulin and glucose interactions in nondiabetic men," *Metabolism*, 1994; 43(5): 599-603. *Also:* Marin, P. et al., "The effects of testosterone treatment on body composition and metabolism in middle-aged obese men," *International Journal of Obesity*, 1992; 16: 991-997.

17. McCullly, K. S., "Homocysteine metabolism in scurvy, growth and arteriosclerosis," *Nature*, 1971; 231: 391-392.

Chapter 8

1. Morgentaler, A. et al., "Occult prostate cancer in men with low serum testosterone levels," *Journal of the American Medical Association*, 1995; 276(23).

2. Carter, H. B. et al., "Longitudinal evaluation of serum androgen levels in men with and without prostate cancer," *The Prostate*, 1995; 27: 25-31.

3. Monath, J. R. et al., "Physiologic variations of serum testosterone within the normal range do not affect serum prostate specific antigen," *Urology*, 1995; 46(l): 58-61. *See also:* Monda, J. M. et al., "The correlation between serum prostate specific antigen and prostate cancer is not influenced by the serum testosterone concentration," *Urology*, 1995; 46(l): 62-64.

4. Suzuki, K. et al., "Endocrine environment of benign prostatic hyperplasia: prostate size and volume are correlated with serum estrogen concentration," *Scandanavian Journal of Urology and Nephrology*, 1995; 29: 65-68. *See also:* Gann, P. H. et al., "A prospective study of plasma hormone levels, nonhormonal factors, and development of benign prostatic hyperplasia," *The Prostate*, 1995; 26: 40-49.

5. Ettinger, B. et al., "Reduced mortality associated with long-term post-menopausal estrogen therapy," *Obstetrics and Gynecology*, 1996; 87: 6-12.

6. Ghanadian, R. and Puah, C. M., "The clinical significance of steroid hormone measurements in the management of patients with prostatic cancer," *World Journal of Urology*, 1983; 1: 49-54. *See also:* Geller, J. et al., "DHT concentrations in human prostate cancer tissue," *Journal of Clinical Endocrinology and Metabolism*, 1978; 46: 440-444. *Also:* Gustafsson, O. et al., "Dihydrotestosterone and testostserone levels in men screened for prostate cancer: a study of a randomized population," *British Journal of Urology*, 1996; 77: 133-140.

Chapter 9

1. Cooper, C. and Campion, G., "Hip fractures in the elderly: a worldwide projection," *Osteoporosis International*, 1992; 2: 285-289.

2. Baran, D. T., "Effect of testosterone therapy on bone formation in an osteoporotic hypogonadal male," *Calcified Tissue Research*, 1978; 26: 103-106.

3. Murphy, S. et al., "Sex hormones and bone mineral density in elderly men," *Bone Mineral*, 1993; 20: 133-140. *See also:* Jackson, J. A. et al., "Testosterone deficiency as a risk factor for hip fractures in men: a case-control study," *American Journal of Medical Science*, 1992; 304: 4-8. *Also:* Stanley, H. L. et al., "Does hypogonadism contribute to the occurence of a minimal trauma hip fracture in elderly men?" *Journal of the American Geriatric Society*," 1991; 39: 766-771.

4. Rudman, D. et al., "Relations of endogenous anabolilc hormones and physical activity to bone mineral density and lean body mass in elderly men," *Journal of Clinical Endocrinology*, 1994; 40: 653-661

5. Lemann, J. et al., "Possible role of carbohydrate induced calciura in calcium oxalate kidney stone formation," *New England Journal of Medicine*, 1969; 280: 232-237.

6. Yudkin, J., *Sweet and Dangerous*, Bantam Books, (New York), 1973.

Chapter 10

1. Nabulsi, A. A. et al., "Association of hormone-replacement therapy with various cardiovascular risk factors in postmenopausal women," *New England Journal of Medicine*, 1993; 328: 1069-1075. *See also:* Manson, J. E., "Postmenopausal hormone therapy and atherosclerotic disease," *American Heart Journal*, 1994; 128(6 Pt2): 1337-1343.

2. Stevenson, J. C. et al., "Hormone replacement therapy and the cardiovascular system. Nonlipid effects," *Drugs*, 1994; 47(2): 35-41.

3. Shahar, E. et al., "Relation of hormone-replacement therapy to measures of plasma fibrinolytic activity," *Circulation*, 1996; 93(11): 1970-1975.

4. McEwen, B. S. et al., "Steroid and thyroid hormones modulate a changing brain," *Journal of Steroid Biochemistry and Molecular Biology*, 1991; 40(1-3): 1-14.

5. Henderson, V. W. et al., "Estrogen replacement therapy in older women. Comparisons between Alzheimer's disease cases and nondemented control subjects," *Archives of Neurology*, 1994; 51(9): 896-900.

6. Paganini-Hill, A. and Henderson, V. W., "Estrogen deficiency and risk of Alzheimer's disease in women," *American Journal of Epidemiology*, 1994; 140(3): 256-261.

7. Tang, M. X. et al., "Effect of oestrogen during menopause on risk and age at onset of Alzheimer's disease," *Lancet*, 1996; 348: 429-432.

8. Phillips, S. M. and Sherwin, B. B., "Effects of estrogen on memory function in surgically menopausal women," *Psychoneuroendocrinology*, 1992; 17(5): 485-495.

9. Sand, R. and Studd, J., "Exogenous androgens in postmenopausal women," *American Journal of Medicine*, 1995; 98(1A).

10. Barlow, D. H. et al., "Long-term hormone implant therapy; hormonal and clinical effects," *Obstetrics and Gynecology*, 1986; 67: 321-325.

Chapter 11

1. Rudman, D. et al., "Effects of human growth hormone in men over 60 years old," *New England Journal of Medicine*, 1990; 323: 1-6. *See also:* Vermulen, A. et al., "Influences of some biological indexes on sex hormone–binding globulin and adrogen levels in aging or obese males," *Journal of Clinical Endocrinology and Metabolism*, 1996; 81(5): 1821-1826.

2. Khansari, D. N. and Gustad, T., "Effects of long-term, low-dose growth hormone therapy on immune function and life expectancy of mice," *Mechanisms of Aging and Development*, 1991; 57: 87-100.

3. Crist, D. M. et al., "Exogenous growth hormone treatment alters body composition and increases natural killer cell activity in women with impaired endogenous growth hormone secretion," *Metabolism*, 1987; 36(12): 1115-1117.

4. Aroonsakul, C. "Reduced growth hormone in Alzheimer's disease," *Journal of Advancement in Medicine*, 1995; 8(3): 206-208.

Index